America's #1 C

NATURAL HEALING FOR DOGS AND CATS

By the Editors of *Prevention* Health Books

RODALE

ST. MARTIN'S
PAPERBACKS

If you purchased this book without a cover, you should be aware that this book is stolen property. It was reported as "unsold and destroyed" to the publisher, and neither the author nor the publisher has received any payment for this "stripped book."

Notice
This book is intended as a reference volume only, not as a medical manual. The information given here is designed to help you make informed decisions about your pet's health. It is not intended as a substitute for any treatment that may have been prescribed by your veterinarian. If you suspect that your pet has a medical problem, we urge you to seek competent medical help.

The information in this book is excerpted from *Pet Speak* (Rodale, 2000) *New Choices in Natural Healing for Dogs and Cats* (Rodale, 1999), and *Prevention's Symptom Solver for Dogs and Cats* (Rodale, 1999).

Prevention's Best is a trademark and *Prevention* Health Books is a registered trademark of Rodale Inc.

NATURAL HEALING FOR DOGS AND CATS

© 2001 by Rodale Inc.

Cover Designer: Anne Twomey
Book Designer: Keith Biery

All rights reserved. No part of this book may be used or reproduced in any manner whatsoever without written permission except in the case of brief quotations embodied in critical articles or reviews. For information, address Rodale Inc., 33 East Minor Street, Emmaus, PA 18098.

ISBN 0–312–97878–2   paperback

Printed in the United States of America

Rodale/St. Martin's Paperbacks edition published July 2001

St. Martin's Paperbacks are published by St. Martin's Press, 175 Fifth Avenue, New York, NY 10010.

10 9 8 7 6 5 4 3 2 1

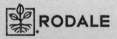

RODALE

WE INSPIRE AND ENABLE PEOPLE TO IMPROVE
THEIR LIVES AND THE WORLD AROUND THEM

Board of Advisors

C. A. Tony Buffington, D.V.M., Ph.D.
Professor of veterinary clinical sciences at the Ohio State University in Columbus

Karen L. Campbell, D.V.M.
Professor of dermatology and endocrinology at the University of Illinois College of Veterinary Medicine at Urbana–Champaign

Liz Palika
A columnist for *Dog Fancy* magazine; owner of the Dog Training with Liz obedience school in Oceanside, California; and author of *All Dogs Need Some Training*

Allen M. Schoen, D.V.M.
Affiliate faculty member in the department of clinical sciences at Colorado State University in Fort Collins; director of the Veterinary Institute for Therapeutic Alternatives in Sherman, Connecticut; and author of *Love, Miracles, and Animal Healing*

John C. Wright, Ph.D.
A certified applied animal behaviorist; professor of psychology at Mercer University in Macon, Georgia; and author of *The Dog Who Would Be King* and *Is Your Cat Crazy?*

Contents

Part Three: Common Behavior Problems

Resources

Introduction

Veterinary medicine used to be much simpler. Without a lot of equipment to lug around, vets made house calls, dispensing medicine along with the wisdom of years of experience. They got to know the families they worked with and had special insights into pets' lives—what they ate, how they spent their days, and what their usual energy was like. They looked at symptoms, too, but only as part of a larger picture.

As technology advanced and veterinarians got more sophisticated, some of this personal touch was lost. Modern vets still depend on good, old-fashioned horse sense but rely more on the latest tests and techniques, like magnetic resonance imaging, keyhole surgery, and computer-designed medications.

For pets with serious injuries, this modern approach is hard to beat, says David H. Jaggar, D.C., M.R.C.V.S. (member of Royal College of Veterinary Surgeons, a British equivalent of D.V.M.), a holistic veterinarian and chiropractor in Boulder, Colorado, and a founder of the International Veterinary Acupuncture Society. It has limitations, however. When owners bring in their pets, some vets focus mainly on the symptoms to prescribe a specific treatment. For instance, a dog with hip dysplasia might be given steroids to relieve swelling and perhaps have surgery done to repair or replace the damaged joint. This relieves the immediate symptom but may not resolve the underlying problems that made the joint vulnerable in the first place, says Dr. Jaggar. And the treatments themselves may cause additional problems.

Veterinarians who specialize in holistic medicine feel that there is a better way. Without rejecting the many advances of modern medicine, they have shifted their focus to an older style of care. They may spend more time with pets in order to understand their personalities and lifestyles. More important, they look at physical and emotional problems as pieces of a larger puzzle. Illness is rarely caused by something as obvious as a weak joint, bacteria in the body, or pollen. In the holistic view, pets get sick because something happened that allowed external factors to cause illness. Unless you strengthen the body, dogs and cats will continue to get sick.

Most illnesses, including such things as allergies, arthritis, diabetes, and even cancer, can be partly controlled—and prevented—by harnessing the body's natural healing powers.

The Search for Answers

Most holistic veterinarians started out as mainstream practitioners. Dr. Jaggar, for example, was on the faculty as a veterinarian at the College of Medicine at the University of Cincinnati. But he, along with many of his colleagues, found himself frustrated because the conventional focus on symptoms didn't seem to work as well as it should.

Along with his colleagues in holistic health, Dr. Jaggar discovered that many natural therapies used in human medicine—like herbs, flower essences, and homeopathy— work just as well for dogs and cats. Unlike drugs, which target specific symptoms, these and other natural remedies tend to have wider-ranging effects—on the emotions, on various organs, and even on the personality, Dr. Jaggar says.

Not all alternative treatments are thousands of years old or come from the ends of the Earth. Holistic veterinarians also use traditional, homegrown cures, such as Kaopectate for diarrhea or peppermint tea for an upset stomach. Herbs often contain the same active ingredients as modern drugs, minus the side effects.

Veterinarians usually study for 8 to 10 years before receiving their D.V.M. (doctor of veterinary medicine) or V.M.D. (veterinariae medicinae doctor) degree. For holistic veterinarians, that is just the beginning. They continue their education by studying such things as acupressure, chiropractic, and homeopathy.

Some veterinary schools and universities offer classes and lectures on alternative medicine, but many of these treatments are still so new that academic instruction may not be available. Holistic veterinarians get most of their training from professional associations, such as the Academy of Veterinary Homeopathy and the International Veterinary Acupuncture Society. Or they apprentice themselves to experts in various fields.

Blended Care

Holistic veterinarians usually specialize in one or more alternative therapies, but they are well-versed in conventional medicine as well. This means that dogs and cats get the best of both worlds—the latest advances in mainstream medicine combined with the safety and effectiveness of natural treatments.

"Holistic care sometimes works better than conventional medicine. Sometimes it works best as a complementary treatment, and sometimes it doesn't work as well but has fewer side effects," says Allen M. Schoen, D.V.M., director of the Veterinary Institute for Therapeutic Alternatives in Sherman, Connecticut, and author of *Love, Miracles, and Animal Healing*.

Dogs and cats with serious illnesses and injuries often receive a blend of treatments—surgery or transfusions, for example, combined with a flower essence like Bach Rescue Remedy to keep the body stable during the trauma. Pets with chronic conditions such as hip pain often do better with holistic care alone.

This blended approach is the reason many people take their pets to holistic veterinarians. They know that they will get the benefits of the latest research, along with time-tested natural treatments. Veterinarians appreciate this versatility as well. They may use conventional medicine to diagnose a bone fracture or detect cancer, then turn to holistic care to help pets recover more quickly. "I once treated a cat with homeopathy before surgically removing a piece of corncob that was stuck in the intestine," says Christina Chambreau, D.V.M., a holistic veterinarian in Sparks, Maryland, and education chairperson for the Academy of Veterinary Homeopathy. "I expected to see severe damage, but the homeopathy helped the abdomen stay healthy, with no inflammation at all."

This book takes the blended approach to pet health. In it, you'll learn how the country's top holistic veterinarians treat their own pets without using drugs—and how you, too, can do it. But you'll also learn which symptoms mean it's time to call a vet and what preventive measures you can take to keep small problems from getting out of hand in the first place. Use this natural healing system to help your pet enjoy lifelong good health.

PART ONE

The Best Choices in Natural Healing

Prevention:
The Best Care

One of the first things we do when we bring home a new pet is find a veterinarian. But your vet spends only an hour or two a year with your pet. He can't be there every day to notice the little changes in your pet's health and behavior that may turn into problems later on. It's up to you to handle all the small things that will keep your pet happy and healthy for the rest of his life.

By watching your pet closely, you will know when trouble is brewing. In this chapter, you will discover ways to keep him from getting sick in the first place. The payoff is tremendous: a small amount of time for a lifetime of love.

Home Safety

Every year, thousands of pets get hurt when their curiosity leads them into dangerous territory. You don't want to stop dogs and cats from exploring, but you do want to keep them safe. Take a few minutes to see things the way they see them—from floor level. Get down on your hands and knees and explore the house, room by room. Look for things that they can reach, chew, or swallow, like string or sewing supplies, says Victoria Valdez, D.V.M., a veterinarian in private practice in Orange, California. Are there cabinets they can nose open or cleaning supplies in paw's reach? The more attractions you can identify—and either move or safely secure—the less likely your pets are to get hurt, she says.

Watch out for electricity. Electrical cords can seem like perfect chew toys—until your pet's sharp teeth penetrate the insulation and hit the wires inside. Dr. Valdez recommends hiding electrical cords under carpets or behind furniture. Or tape them firmly to the floor.

Keep medicines out of reach. Even mild human medicines like acetaminophen can be extremely dangerous for

Which Plants Are Poison?

For dogs and cats, many houseplants and shrubs are poisonous. Among the worst are poinsettias, philodendrons, and dieffenbachias. "There are alkaline chemicals in the leaves of poinsettias that cause gastrointestinal upset," says Robin Downing, D.V.M., a veterinarian in private practice in Windsor, Colorado. Here are a few other plants that you'll want to keep out of reach.

- Amaryllis
- Azalea
- Caladium
- Calla or arum lily
- Daffodil
- Delphinium
- Elephant's ear
- English holly
- Foxglove
- Ivy
- Jade plant
- Jerusalem cherry
- Morning glory
- Mums (pot and spider)
- Privet
- Wisteria

dogs and cats. It's not enough to stash them on top of the bureau or in a partly closed drawer. And a childproof cap won't slow down an inquisitive puppy for more than a minute or two, says Dr. Valdez. So be sure to keep medicines well out of reach or behind tightly closed doors.

Cover the windows. Young pets are attracted to open windows and balconies. Every year, a few unfortunate dogs and cats accidentally tumble from upper stories, causing serious injuries. Make sure that screens fit snugly and are in good repair. If you have a balcony, keep the door to it closed.

Shut the lids on appliances. Vets recommend getting into the habit of closing appliances—including trash compactors, washing machines, and dishwashers—when they're not in use. It's also a good idea to check for visitors before hitting the on switch.

Cover the commode. "If you leave the toilet seat up, it looks like a chair from a kitten's point of view, and she's going to jump up," says Dr. Valdez. For small cats particularly, it's not always easy to get out. "It's porcelain, so they can't get a foothold," she explains.

Do a car check. Cats love to curl up under the hoods of cars because heat from the engine keeps them pleasantly warm. You don't have to open the hood every time you go for a drive. Just rap it soundly with your hand—the noise will drive out guests before the gears and belts start turning, says Dr. Valdez.

Make the garage off-limits. Many chemicals that we use every day, like insecticides and antifreeze, are downright tasty—and deadly—to dogs and cats. It's essential to keep your pets away from danger zones and to keep chemicals off the floor and put away.

Provide some traction. For puppies particularly, slick linoleum floors can be hard to negotiate. And the lack of traction can actually damage his bones and joints. "A rug that won't slip will keep the young puppy from slipping and harming his hip socket, which is still being formed when he's young," says Jim Corbin, Ph.D., professor emeritus of animal nutrition at the University of Illinois in Urbana.

The Home Exam

While annual exams are essential, there are limits to what your vet can learn during a 30-minute visit. Vets recommend doing a complete home exam at least once a month, says Priscilla Stockner, D.V.M., executive director of the Animal Center and Humane Society in Escondido, California. But you don't have to follow a formal plan. Just watch for *anything* that seems different. Here are the main things to cover.

Do an infection inspection. The eyes, ears, and nose are the places most likely to get infected. Signs of infection include a bad odor, redness, swelling, or a discharge, says Robin Downing, D.V.M., a veterinarian in private practice in Windsor, Colorado.

Check for mites. Ear mites are tiny parasites that can cause intense itching and, sometimes, infections in the ear canal. Look at the wax in your pet's ears. It should be light or dark yellow. If it's black or brown and gritty-looking, he probably has mites, and you will want to take care of them.

Monitor his weight. It's normal for pets to gain a little weight as they get older. If your dog or cat has suddenly put on a lot of weight—or if he has suddenly started to lose weight—call your vet.

Look for lumps. Many dogs and cats develop lumps under the skin. Unfortunately, there's no way to tell at home if a lump is harmless or not, so it's essential to call your vet if a new one develops. This is especially true of cats since they are more likely than dogs to develop cancerous lumps.

Does the Nose Know?

A warm nose doesn't mean your dog's sick, any more than a cool, wet nose means he's healthy. "I've seen pets with high temperatures that have cold, wet noses," says Robin Downing, D.V.M., a veterinarian in private practice in Windsor, Colorado. "The temperature of the nose isn't a very reliable measure of an animal's wellness."

The only way to check your pet's temperature is the old-fashioned way: by using a rectal thermometer.

Looking Good, Feeling Good

Regular grooming is a great way to find problems you might otherwise miss—fleas in the fur, for example, or small bumps on the skin. Vets have even found that regular grooming can help prevent a variety of health problems. Here is what they advise.

Brush them often. Brushing your dog or cat distributes natural oils over your pet's skin, which can help prevent rashes and infections. For cats, brushing is important because it reduces the amount of hair they swallow—and invariably cough up later as a hair ball. Short-haired pets can be brushed once a week. For dogs and cats with longer fur, a daily brushing will help keep them healthy and looking good.

Go after mats. Mats trap moisture next to the skin, making it easier for bacteria or parasites to thrive, says John Hamil, D.V.M., a veterinarian in private practice in Laguna Beach, California. Hair mats are tricky to remove because the skin underneath is often tender. If you can convince your pet to hold still, you can often work out mats using a brush and comb, says Virginia Parker Guidry, grooming columnist for *Dog Fancy* magazine. To make things easier, she recommends a detangler spray, available in pet supply stores. If the mat is too tight to remove or if it is right against the skin, you may have to clip it out with a pair of blunt-nosed scissors. Clip carefully so as not to nick the skin.

Do a "pet-icure." Your pet's nails are constantly growing. Trim them regularly so they don't crack or tear, says Dr. Valdez. Have your vet show you how.

Keep his teeth clean. Brushing several times a week—or, better yet, every day—will help keep teeth clean and bacteria-free. Vets have found that the same bacteria in the mouth that cause gum disease can get into the bloodstream, possibly damaging the heart or other organs.

Fighting Fleas

Fleas are more than just itchy. They also transmit tapeworm, which can cause diarrhea or other intestinal problems. Controlling fleas is an important part of keeping your pet healthy, says John Hamil, D.V.M., a veterinarian in private practice in Laguna Beach, California.

One strategy is to use an oral medication such as Program. Given monthly, this prescription drug stops fleas from reproducing on your pet. It doesn't affect dogs and cats, but it does cause the flea population to plunge. Your vet may also recommend products that, when applied to the animal's coat, kill fleas directly. Used in combination with an oral medication, such products can help eliminate fleas for good, says Dr. Hamil.

When you are ready to wage war on fleas, it is essential to clean the house thoroughly, especially in areas where your pet spends his time. Washing his bedding in hot water will help kill fleas as well as their eggs, stopping the flea cycle at the source.

Don't forget the ears. The ears don't require much care beyond regular inspections for ear mites. But you can periodically swab out the outer portions of the ears with a dry cotton ball. Or your vet may recommend using a combination ear cleaner/disinfectant. Don't use cotton swabs to clean out the ear canal since this can push wax and debris in, Dr. Stockner warns.

Homeward Bound

Using identification tags is perhaps the most effective (and least expensive) way of keeping your pet safe, says Dr. Stockner. Tags should have your name and phone number. (With cats, some people go one step further and include a line that says, "If I'm outside, I'm lost.") Veterinarians advise against putting your pet's name on his tag because that could make it easier for thieves to lure him away.

For additional protection, ask your vet about tattoos or microchips. Tags often get lost, but tattoos are permanent. The same is true of microchips, which are implanted beneath the skin, usually between the shoulder blades. If your pet gets lost and doesn't have his tags, a veterinarian or animal shelter will still be able to identify him. Used together, tags, tattoos, and microchips help ensure that a lost friend finds his way home again.

The Kindest Cut

Spaying and neutering are among the cheapest, most effective strategies for preventing a number of serious health threats.

In males, neutering involves removing the testicles. This is important because in unneutered males the prostate gland typically enlarges with age, starting when a dog is 6 or 7 years old. If the gland gets too large, it can begin pressing on the urethra, making it difficult to uri-nate. Unneutered males are also at risk for prostate infec-tions, along with testicular cancer, says Peggy Rucker, D.V.M., a veterinarian in private practice in Lebanon, Virginia.

As a behavioral bonus, neutering males also makes them much less likely to roam or get in fights with other pets. "An intact male cat's life span is about half that of a neutered cat's," adds Dr. Rucker.

When female pets are spayed, the uterus and ovaries are removed. This completely eliminates the risk of uterine infections and substantially reduces the risk of breast cancer, Dr. Rucker says.

Veterinarians recommend neutering pets when they are about 6 months old, although it can be done earlier or later. Generally, younger pets recover more quickly and are back to normal in a day or two, says W. Marvin Mackie, D.V.M., a veterinarian in private practice in the Los Angeles area.

Exercising for Total Health

Puppies and kittens bounce off the walls as if they had springs on the bottoms of their feet. Their high energy may drive you nuts at times, but it is a natural leftover from life on the wild side, when it prepared furry babies for survival as adults.

Today, of course, many dogs and cats happily spend their leisure time snoozing on the sofa or lounging on windowsills. About one in three dogs and cats is overweight because of lack of exercise. Overweight pets are prone to joint problems because the joints don't stay lubricated. They have behavior problems since pets without outlets for their energy are more likely to become aggressive, frustrated, or destructive, says Wayne Hunthausen, D.V.M., a veterinary behaviorist in Westwood, Kansas, and coauthor of *Handbook of Behaviour Problems of the Dog and Cat*.

Holistic veterinarians and their mainstream counterparts now believe that regular exercise is among the most important tools for keeping pets healthy, both physically and emotionally, says Ihor Basko, D.V.M., a holistic veterinarian in private practice in Honolulu and Kilauea, Hawaii. Dogs and cats that exercise regularly live up to 30 percent longer than those that don't. They have stronger lungs and hearts, and they have more energy. Regular exercise can even reverse health problems. In one study, dogs with congestive heart failure exercised for 2 hours a day. Four weeks later, their hearts were significantly healthier when compared with dogs that didn't move their furry tails. Veterinarians have even found that exercise may play a role in healing nerve damage, allowing some pets with paralysis to walk again.

Exercise allows food to be digested more completely, which means that there is less waste in the body to put a strain on the kidneys, says Kathleen Carson, D.V.M., a holistic veterinarian in private practice in Hermosa Beach, California. On an emotional level, exercise reduces boredom, frustration, and aggression. It stimulates the mind so that dogs and cats stay interested in life, says Mary Lee Nitschke, Ph.D., professor of psychology at Linfield College in Portland, Oregon, and an animal behaviorist in Beaverton.

For most pets, a romp in the backyard, a walk around the block, or running up and down the stairs does the trick. Dogs and cats should exercise 20 to 40 minutes twice a day, says Dr. Basko. But it doesn't have to be the same routine every day. You could go for a walk in the morning, then play in the backyard in the evening. Or jog one day and swim the next. Of course, every pet is different, so you should ask your vet to help you plan an exercise program that's right for yours.

Walking

The single best exercise for pets is walking. Going for walks releases energy and flexes and strengthens the

Puppy Precautions

Puppies have energy levels that can leave their owners gasping for air. It seems logical that vigorous exercise would be the perfect way to cool their exuberance a bit. But too much exercise can injure their growth plates (the areas near joints that generate new bone) and interfere with their normal growth.

Dogs mature at different rates, so there are different guidelines for every breed. As a rule, small breeds (full-grown weight of under 25 pounds) can handle vigorous exercise once they reach 8 months; larger dogs (adult weight of 45 to 90 pounds) shouldn't take long walks or runs until they are about 12 months old, and giant breeds should take it easy until they are 18 months old.

joints. And it works well for pets of all ages, says Anne Lampru, D.V.M., a holistic veterinarian in private practice in Tampa, Florida.

Walking isn't ideal for cats, of course, unless you are willing to spend time training them to accept a harness and lead. And it is not always the best choice for big dogs since they may tend to walk you rather than the other way around. But for most dogs—and for cats, as long as you are walking around the yard or up and down stairs—walking is about your best choice. Here is what veterinarians advise.

Get your pet breathing hard. A leisurely walk is better than no walk at all, but your pet will get the most benefits when you go fast enough and long enough to get him breathing hard. For most pets, a 20-minute walk twice a day is about right, says Dr. Basko. Of course, an energetic dog needs to cover more ground than an older, slower pet. And pets that are out of shape may find a 20-minute walk a little too much at first. So start slowly until your pet is comfortable going farther and faster.

For pets that haven't been exercising regularly, start with 5 minutes of exercise three to five times a week, then slowly increase the exercise until they are getting 20 to 60 minutes a day, says Susan G. Wynn, D.V.M., a veterinarian in Atlanta and coeditor of *Complementary and Alternative Veterinary Medicine*. If your pet has been ill or is seriously out of shape, talk to your vet before you start exercising him regularly, she adds.

Dogs are often more interested in smelling—and wetting—the roses than just walking past them, so you may have to struggle a bit to keep your pet moving. You will know that you are moving fast enough when his breathing rate speeds up and stays elevated for most of the walk. Panting won't hurt him, but be prepared to slow down if he struggles to get his breath, is slowing down, or simply sits down and refuses to move. Let him rest for a few minutes before moving on, says Dr. Nitschke.

Small dogs can often get by with shorter walks than large ones can, simply because their short legs have to move pretty fast to keep up with your normal stride. So don't be surprised when a dog such as a toy poodle is ready to go home sooner than a golden retriever, says Dr. Nitschke.

Work around his schedule. No one wants to exercise after a big meal, dogs and cats included. It is best to take dogs and cats for walks before meals, says Dr. Nitschke. And once you get outside, be prepared to stop a few times while they make pit stops. Most pets will take care of their business in the first few minutes, so you can walk pretty steadily after that.

Plan for the weather. Dogs and cats can't take off their coats the way you can, and temperatures that feel comfortable to you may be uncomfortably warm for them.

When the humidity or temperature is high, walk more slowly than usual and be prepared to go home early.

You need to be especially cautious if you have a bulldog or another breed with a short, pushed-in face. They don't breathe as efficiently as other dogs and have a higher risk of getting heatstroke, says Dr. Hunthausen.

Where you walk also makes a difference. Concrete sidewalks can get hot even on relatively mild days. Your pet's foot pads provide a lot of protection, but they aren't proof against scorching heat, says Dr. Carson.

Winter causes its own problems, Dr. Carson adds. Air that is colder than about 20°F is hard on the lungs. In addition, your pet's paw pads won't protect him from constant moisture, road salt, or sharp shards of ice.

Many winter walkers invest in a stout pair of booties for their pets, available in pet supply stores. Booties are very effective at protecting the paws, but most dogs don't like wearing them; they are often more trouble than they are worth, says Dr. Nitschke. Sweaters, however, are another story. Short-haired pets like Chihuahuas are especially vulnerable to winter's chill and enjoy having an extra layer of comfort, she adds.

Vary the routine. Dogs and cats love new sights, smells, and sounds, and they get bored if you walk the same route every day. Walking in different directions and neighborhoods or even in different parts of a park helps keep them interested. In fact, you will get more exercise bang for your buck when you change routes because pets get more enthusiastic when they are going someplace new, says Dr. Nitschke.

Swimming

Walking is the most convenient exercise, but for pets that like water, swimming is hard to beat. It works almost every muscle in the body, and the buoyancy of the water reduces stress on the legs and back. Pets that are overweight or have arthritis or previous injuries can often swim with no discomfort at all, says Donn W. Griffith, D.V.M., a holistic veterinarian in private practice in Dublin, Ohio.

Big dogs need quite a bit of water to swim comfortably, so it may be hard to find a good place to take them, adds Kathy Kern, a registered veterinary technician and owner of Animal Fitness Center at Almaden Valley Animal Hospital in San Jose, California. Small pets, on the other hand, may be able to do laps in your bathtub.

Since many dogs (and even some cats) take naturally to water, you don't have to worry about giving them swimming lessons. You do have to make sure, however, that they are comfortable as well as safe.

Stick to warm-water swimming. Even though cold-climate breeds like Labradors don't object to frigid water, the

The Healing Instinct

Pets experience stress just like people do. A change in your schedule, workers in the house, or a neighbor's dog visiting the yard can put their tails in a twist. Too much stress can weaken the immune system and cause a host of emotional and physical problems, says Michael W. Fox, B.V.M. (bachelor of veterinary medicine, a British equivalent of D.V.M.), Ph.D., a veterinary consultant in Washington, D.C., and author of *The Healing Touch*.

When stress levels rise, dogs and cats instinctively try to blow off steam—and their favorite way to do it is with vigorous play. A few minutes' running around stimulates their minds, defuses frustration, and helps keep them emotionally and physically fit, Dr. Fox explains.

cold causes muscles to tighten and contract, which can lead to injuries if you aren't careful, Kern says. Ponds, swimming pools, and even the ocean are fine as long as the outside temperature is warm, she adds. For small pets that are swimming in the tub, the water should be between 85° and 90°F.

Give some support. Pets that don't swim well or are recovering from health problems may need a little help staying afloat, Kern says. She recommends gently holding the base of the tail while your pet paddles away from you. He won't make any progress, but he won't know this, and swimming in place is excellent exercise, she says. It also ensures that he won't bash into the sides of the tub or pool.

Limit his exertion. Swimming is vigorous exercise, and pets that aren't used to it will get sore if you let them go too long. Kern recommends letting your pet swim for 5 to 10 minutes two days in a row. This will loosen up stiffness and get his muscles in shape. As time goes by, you can let him swim for longer periods. For most pets, though, 10 to 20 minutes is plenty, she says.

Rinse him well. Chlorine, ocean salt, and other things in water can irritate the skin. And pond scum will perfume your house for days at a time. It is worth hosing off your dog right after his swim. Dry him well and dab excess water from inside the ears to help prevent infections, Dr. Hunthausen says.

Fun and Games

Every exercise plan should include plenty of planned playtime. It is especially important for cats since play is often the main way they exercise, says Dr. Griffith. As with any form of exercise, games should be fast-paced and vigorous enough to get your pet's heart and lungs working for about 20 minutes at a stretch.

You can find all kinds of toys at pet supply stores, but it is easy to make your own. You may not even need any toys at all. Cats, for example, often love chasing the covers when you are making the bed. You can make a real game out of it if you want to. And dogs—especially terriers—really dig digging. The next time your dog shows an interest in helping you garden, hide a few treats in his personal patch of ground and watch the dirt fly. He will get a great workout, and all you have to do is sit back and smile.

Every dog and cat enjoys different kinds of games, but here are some common favorites.

Catch. Almost all dogs—and even some cats, especially Siamese—love chasing things, although they are not always interested in bringing them back, says Dr. Griffith. It is pretty hard to go wrong tossing a tennis ball, a ball of string, or a catnip mouse. Just be sure that whatever you are throwing is too big for your pet to swallow and that it doesn't have sharp edges or splinters.

Herding games. Some dog breeds, like corgis and Border collies, are bred for herding. One way to keep them entertained is with a boomer ball. This is a large rubber ball that dogs can bump, bite, and bully all over the yard.

Keep-away. Cats and some terriers love games of chase and capture. Pet stores sell fishing pole toys, with which you cast a furry lure across your pet's line of sight. But it is just as easy to put a feather or a piece of fabric on the end of a string and toss it around, says Dr. Lampru. Just be sure to let him catch it periodically to keep him from getting frustrated, she adds. In addition, cats have a hard time detecting objects that are coming straight toward them, so always draw the string and lure across his line of sight.

Hide-and-seek. Dogs adore a good treasure hunt, with food as the treasure. Take some of your dog's favorite treats and stash them around the house—under a book, leaning against a table leg, or under a corner of the carpet. Lead him to one treat so he gets the idea, then relax while his nose goes to work. Some dogs will search for food by the hour, says Dr. Hunthausen. You can play a variation of this game by getting your dog a toy such as the Buster Cube or Goody Ship. These toys have hidden compartments that you fill with food. The food comes out a little at a time, so dogs have to nose, nudge, and shake them around to get their reward.

King of the mountain. Get your cat moving by taking advantage of his natural inclination to climb to high places. Put his favorite toy or a tasty tidbit in a high place—on top of a bookcase or, for out-of-shape cats, midway up the stairs—so that he has to jump or climb to get it.

Old-Fashioned
Home Remedies

Dogs and cats have more exuberance than common sense. Their full-speed-ahead enthusiasm makes them a lot of fun, but it also leaves them throwing up after they gobble pilfered snacks or hobbling with cuts or bruises when they run without looking. Which is why most owners, sooner or later, discover the value of old-fashioned care.

Some pet problems always require a trip to the vet, but the majority can be handled at home, says Michelle Tilghman, D.V.M., a holistic veterinarian in private practice in Stone Mountain, Georgia. In fact, many old-fashioned home treatments are the same ones that veterinarians use, and for good reason: They work.

Consider ice. Nothing complicated about it, but it is still one of the best remedies for relieving pain and reducing swelling and inflammation. Vinegar is another one. Vets use it all the time for treating skin problems, although they usually call it acetic acid, just to be fancy. Even remedies as simple as herbal teas and cool-water rinses can work as well as modern medications.

One reason veterinarians feel comfortable recommending old-fashioned treatments is that research has shown they work. In fact, many traditional remedies contain ingredients that are similar to those used in modern drugs and treatments. Warm milk, for example, calms pets down and helps them sleep, says Mary Lee Nitschke, Ph.D., professor of psychology at Linfield College in Portland, Oregon, and an animal behaviorist in Beaverton. That's because it contains the amino acid tryptophan, which is converted in the brain to a chemical that tells the body when to rest.

One of the best things about old-fashioned care is that many treatments use ingredients you already have. Suppose, for example, your dog has a hot spot. This painful skin infection can spread within hours. You could rush to your vet for a hot-spot remedy. Or you could moisten a tea bag and apply it to the spot. Tea contains tannic acid, a natural astringent that dries hot spots and helps them heal, says Lowell Ackerman, D.V.M., a veterinary dermatologist in Mesa, Arizona, and author of the *Guide to Skin and Haircoat Problems in Dogs*.

For some illnesses, of course, old-fashioned care isn't going to work. But since you are taking care of your pet yourself, you will know very soon whether or not you need to call your veterinarian. Some holistic vets are happy to give information over the telephone as long as your pet is one of their regular patients. This means that you get the best of both worlds: the natural effectiveness and safety of home care and advice from an expert when you need it most, says Deborah C. Mallu, D.V.M, a holistic veterinarian in private practice in Sedona, Arizona.

How to Use Old-Fashioned Care

Home remedies are very safe compared with drugs, but there are limits to what you can do at home, says Pat

Zook, D.V.M., a holistic veterinarian in private practice in Stone Mountain, Georgia. A little Kaopectate may ease diarrhea after your dog has raided the trash but won't fight salmonella or parvovirus. "Most of the time, pets can fight off a mild infection or injury. But if they are totally overwhelmed, they're going to need treatments only your vet can give," she says. Call your vet when your pet doesn't get better—or starts getting worse—within a day or two

A Strong Defense

Your pet's immune system is designed to destroy most germs that it comes into contact with. But when the immune system doesn't work as well as it should, germs get a dangerous advantage.

Researchers have spent decades and billions of dollars in the search for germ-killing drugs and treatments. But one of the most powerful germ fighters is also one of the oldest: common household bleach.

Unlike antiseptics, which are applied to the skin, disinfectants like bleach are used to clean floors, litter boxes, and other places where germs thrive. When your pet has been ill with ringworm, for example, treating the environment is just as important as treating the disease, says Robert Kennis, D.V.M., a veterinary dermatologist at Texas A&M University College of Veterinary Medicine in College Station. That's because it is the only way to stop him from getting reinfected.

Veterinarians like bleach because it is inexpensive and works against almost every kind of germ. They recommend diluting 1 part bleach in 10 parts water and using the solution to wash bedding and food and water bowls and to wipe down hard surfaces where your pet spends his time.

or when the problem goes away and then comes back, says Dr. Zook.

Even when your pet is being treated by your vet, there is still a place for home remedies, Dr. Zook adds. For most conditions that dogs and cats get, like diarrhea, itching, or cut paw pads, they need a little support as much as they need medical treatment. Nutrition is especially important because pets that are sick tend to lose their appetites, which means they don't get all the nutrients they need to keep the immune system strong.

Veterinarians sometimes use drugs like diazepam (Valium) to stimulate the appetite, says Dr. Zook, but a simpler, safer strategy is to brew up some chicken or beef broth. Even a drizzle of the broth provides essential vitamins and minerals.

Something as simple as hand-feeding will often encourage pets to eat, adds Alice Wolf, D.V.M., professor of medicine at Texas A&M University College of Veterinary Medicine in College Station.

Old-fashioned care tends to work best for digestive complaints, some skin problems, and minor skin infections—conditions that come on suddenly or within a few days. When you know what to do, most of these problems will clear up almost as quickly as they appeared, says Dr. Zook.

Treating Digestive Problems

Most of the time you can clear up bouts of diarrhea and vomiting with simple home remedies like these.

Yogurt. It's one of the best medicines for stopping diarrhea. Live-culture yogurt contains beneficial bacteria that aid in digestion and help keep harmful intestinal bacteria in check, explains Roger L. DeHaan, D.V.M., a holistic veterinarian in private practice in Frazee, Minnesota.

Petroleum jelly. This versatile remedy lubricates the intestines, which is especially helpful for hair balls. In fact, it works better than some commercial hair-ball remedies, which often contain artificial flavors and preservatives, says James R. Richards, D.V.M., director of the Cornell Feline Health Center at Cornell University in Ithaca, New York.

Kaopectate. This medicine-cabinet staple contains a mineral found in clay called attapulgite, coats the digestive tract, and absorbs toxins that cause diarrhea. It is not just a home remedy, adds H. Ellen Whiteley, D.V.M., a veterinary consultant in Guadalupita, New Mexico, and consultant for *The Country Vet's Home Remedies for Cats.* Most veterinarians use it, too.

Fiber. Found in generous amounts in products such as Metamucil and in grains, bran, fresh vegetables, and canned pumpkin, dietary fiber is a superb digestive aid that can relieve constipation and diarrhea, says Dr. Whiteley.

Treating Skin Problems

The skin shields dogs and cats from the elements. It regulates temperature and protects against viruses, bacteria, and environmental toxins. It takes quite a beating, and it is a testimony to skin's toughness that serious problems don't occur more often. But minor skin problems are fairly common, says Dr. Ackerman. Cuts, scrapes, and other irritations occur from time to time. And some dogs and cats suffer from itching a lot more than people do.

Most skin problems are easy to treat at home, says Dr. Ackerman. In fact, many old-fashioned remedies, such as the following, work as well as their medicinal counterparts.

Oatmeal. It's an excellent remedy for itching caused by dry skin, allergies, and insect bites and stings, says Carolyn

The Healing Instinct

Water is one of nature's most potent remedies. Dogs and cats know instinctively that it makes them feel good. For example, dogs that have been bitten by ants or stung by bees often lie in a puddle of water or plaster their bellies against wet grass. In the wild, wolves and moose know instinctively that the quickest way to get away from fleas or flies is to stand neck-deep in the nearest water, and some dogs do the same thing. So if your pet suddenly makes a run for the nearest mud puddle or pool of water, he's just trying to make himself feel better.

Blakey, D.V.M., a holistic veterinarian in private practice in Richmond, Indiana. You can make your own skin soother by filling a cotton sock with rolled oats and running water through it. Or you can use colloidal oatmeal (like Aveeno), which has been ground to a powder so it dissolves in water.

Oil. Safflower and olive oils are easily absorbed by the skin and are good for treating small areas of dryness and irritation. Many vets recommend using oil to relieve chapped noses or cracked paw pads, says Joanne Stefanatos, D.V.M., a holistic veterinarian in private practice in Las Vegas. Hand creams that contain lanolin, a natural oil that comes from sheep's wool, are also good moisturizers.

Ammonia. It doesn't smell pretty, but it is one of the best remedies for insect bites and stings. A number of commercial products, like After Bite, use ammonia as the active ingredient.

Heating pads and cold packs. They're a safe alternative to aspirin (which can be toxic for cats) and other drugs.

Veterinarians often recommend using cold to relieve the pain of bruises and pulled muscles. Heat is one of the best ways to ease long-term problems like painful joints. Hot and cold treatments can be as simple as a washcloth filled with ice, or a hot-water bottle.

Water. It's one of the best remedies for itchy skin, says Allen M. Schoen, D.V.M., director of the Veterinary Institute for Therapeutic Alternatives in Sherman, Connecticut, and author of *Love, Miracles, and Animal Healing*. A cool-water rinse or bath moisturizes the skin and soothes the nerve endings.

Stopping Infections

Veterinarians often use creams or oral medications to kill infection-causing germs, but medications are used mainly only after pets are sick. Holistic veterinarians feel that it makes more sense to strengthen the immune system so it is better able to resist germs before they multiply. Even when dogs and cats do get infections or when they have a high risk of getting one, such as after an injury, you can usually protect them with traditional home care. Here are some home remedies for skin infections.

Soap and water. Simple soaps kill most germs, and the suds and flushing action wash the rest away. You don't need an antibacterial soap. In fact, you may not want one because these soaps are often too harsh, says Steven A. Melman, V.M.D., a veterinarian with practices in Potomac, Maryland, and Palm Springs, California, and author of *Skin Diseases of Dogs and Cats*.

Saline solution. The same stuff that you use to rinse contact lenses is perfect for flushing the eyes and ears and for rinsing wounds. Saline doesn't sting like plain water because its composition is similar to the body's natural fluids.

Vinegar. It contains a mild acid that inhibits the growth of yeast and other organisms that cause infection as well as those that cause dandruff or an oily coat, says Anne Lampru, D.V.M., a holistic veterinarian in private practice in Tampa, Florida. Vinegar also works as an ear cleaner and rinse. Many commercial ear cleansers contain vinegar.

Hydrogen peroxide. This old-fashioned remedy can be a helpful antiseptic for dental care, says Ihor Basko, D.V.M., a holistic veterinarian in private practice in Honolulu and Kilauea, Hawaii. Wetting a toothbrush with two or three drops of hydrogen peroxide and dipping it in baking soda makes a very effective toothpaste, he says.

Isopropyl alcohol. This antiseptic kills germs quickly. It is really too harsh to apply to cuts or scrapes, says Dr. Lampru. But when your pet has been sick and can't tolerate any more problems, you can use alcohol, along with soap and hot water, to sterilize food bowls, kennel floors, and other things that your pet comes in contact with.

Aloe vera juice. This helps wounds heal. First, disinfect cuts and scrapes by spritzing the area forcefully with clean water to remove surface debris. Follow with a spray made from 6 ounces of aloe vera juice and 8 ounces of saline solution or distilled water.

Using the New
Natural Medicines

Modern veterinary medicine has made it possible for dogs and cats to live healthier lives than ever before. Conditions such as diabetes and thyroid disease can now be treated with inexpensive medications. Long-term problems like hip dysplasia are eased with over-the-counter drugs, and most infections can be cured almost instantly with antibiotics.

Conventional drugs, however, aren't perfect solutions. While they are very effective at targeting specific symptoms, they often cause additional problems at the same time. "Aspirin is great at relieving pain, but it can also lead to gastric ulcers and stomach bleeding," says Randy Caviness, D.V.M., clinical instructor of small animal acupuncture at Tufts University School of Veterinary Medicine in North Grafton, Massachusetts, and a holistic veterinarian in private practice in Concord.

A bigger problem is that modern drugs often treat symptoms rather than the underlying causes of disease, says Christina Chambreau, D.V.M., a holistic veterinarian in Sparks, Maryland, and education chairperson for the

Academy of Veterinary Homeopathy. Holistic veterinarians believe there is a better way. They have discovered that natural medicines and techniques like homeopathy and flower essence therapy can strengthen the body so that it is more resistant to disease. At the same time, many of these "new" medicines will stop symptoms just as effectively as drugs—usually without the side effects.

It is not that holistic veterinarians don't use modern medications—most of them do. But by using natural remedies whenever possible, says Dr. Chambreau, you can keep your pets healthier so that they don't need drugs in the first place.

Getting Started

Natural medicines are very safe and easy to use, but they have to be used responsibly, says Michelle Tilghman, D.V.M., a holistic veterinarian in private practice in Stone Mountain, Georgia. Every pet responds differently to various remedies, she explains. It's important to talk to your veterinarian before starting a natural treatment program at home.

It is not always easy to find an expert who can help you choose the best natural remedies and provide instructions on using them safely. Ask your veterinarian (or friends who are already using natural remedies) to recommend an expert trained in homeopathic, herbal, and nutritional medicine. Or you can write to one of the holistic veterinary associations listed on page 261 to locate experts in your area.

Homeopathy: Helping the Body Help Itself

One of the most exciting natural therapies—and one you can start using right away—is homeopathy. Homeopathic medicine is based on the concept that like cures like. The idea is to give pets minuscule amounts of substances that in larger doses would cause the same symptoms as the disease the pet already has. According to experts, this amplifies the original symptom and "wakes up" the body's defenses, allowing them to recognize the problem and gear up for the attack.

When you read the label on a homeopathic remedy, you will see a designation like "1X." This means that the remedy is diluted 1:10, or one part of the active ingredient to nine parts liquid (usually distilled water or alcohol). A dose of 3X means that a remedy has been diluted 1:10 three times. In homeopathy, this is a pretty concentrated dose. Many remedies are 1C, meaning they have been diluted 100 times, or 1M, which have been diluted 1,000 times.

Some researchers speculate that the active ingredients in homeopathic remedies are so minute that they are able to slip through the body's blood–brain barrier, possibly influencing the nervous system in ways that can't be measured yet. "We can't explain exactly how it works, but it is powerful medicine," says Dr. Chambreau.

Putting It to Work

Drugs are generally effective no matter who is taking them, but homeopathic remedies require more of an individualized approach. For instance, a remedy called Nux vomica is often used to treat diarrhea caused by eating rich food. When the diarrhea is caused by something else, the preferred remedy might be Arsenicum. It often takes some trial and error before matching the right remedy with each pet, Dr. Chambreau says.

Homeopathic medicines don't always work quickly, she adds. Short-term problems like diarrhea may get better after giving your pet just a few homeopathic doses. Long-term conditions like arthritis often require long treatments because it takes time for the body to mobilize its defenses.

For simple problems like a sore paw or a runny nose, it is perfectly safe to follow the instructions in this or other books and do homeopathy yourself at home. "Even if you give the wrong remedy by mistake, it is not likely to do harm," adds Russell Swift, D.V.M., a holistic veterinarian in private practice in Dade, Broward, and Palm Beach Counties in Florida.

You can buy homeopathic remedies at health food stores and some pet supply stores. It is fine to use human homeopathic remedies for pets, says Teresa Fulp, D.V.M., a holistic veterinarian in private practice in Springfield, Virginia. "Your pet's size makes absolutely no difference in the amount you give," she adds. "All that matters is how frequently you give it. Giving it more often makes it stronger."

Homeopathic remedies can be expensive. But since the doses are very small and the unused portions last nearly forever, you get a lot of medicine for your money. A good way to begin is to pick up a "home kit," which will include several remedies, along with instructions on using them. When you are just getting started, here is what holistic veterinarians advise.

Try one thing at a time. Even though dogs and cats often have more than one symptom when they are ill, you should use only one remedy at a time. Using too many remedies may interfere with healing, says Dr. Fulp. This is especially true when you are using a remedy blend, she adds. Don't give your pet additional remedies—including nonhomeopathic treatments like flower essences or acupressure—unless your vet tells you to.

Watch for results. While most short-term problems like vomiting or swelling go away on their own, they may clear up more quickly when they are treated with homeopathic remedies. "If your pet isn't feeling better within 2 to 3 days, you have probably chosen the wrong remedy, and you should call your vet," says Dr. Fulp.

Give less instead of more. Unlike drugs, which are designed to knock out symptoms entirely, homeopathic remedies are meant only to help the body heal itself. In most cases, you give the remedy for a day or two, then stand back while your pet's natural healing powers go to work.

Handle them carefully. Homeopathic remedies can lose their power when they are exposed to electromagnetic fields, such as those produced by television sets or even your body. Touching the medicine with your hands can reduce its potency or, if it is absorbed through your skin, affect you more than your pet, says Dr. Fulp. You don't want to hide homeopathic remedies inside treats, either. They must be given without any "sugar coating," she explains. And don't feed your pet within 15 minutes of giving a remedy.

Keep them pure. Homeopathic remedies may lose their effectiveness when they are exposed to heat or sunlight or if they are stored near strong-smelling substances like coffee or perfume. When stored carefully—preferably in a dark, cool place—they retain their potency just about forever, says Dr. Fulp.

Herbs: Nature's Drugs

We often think of herbs as being old-fashioned, but a large percentage of today's medicines are actually derived from their herbal counterparts. Even when herbs contain almost the same chemicals as modern drugs, they are sometimes more effective because they haven't been whittled down to a single component. Willow bark (*Salix alba*), for example, contains a chemical very similar to aspirin, making it an effective pain remedy, says Dr. Caviness. And other things in the willow bark help protect against gastric ulcers, a major side effect of aspirin therapy, he says.

Holistic veterinarians have found that most herbs contain veritable pharmacies of active ingredients within their seeds, roots, leaves, and bark. This means that one herb may be used for many conditions. For instance, slippery elm (*Ulmus rubra*) contains natural compounds that can help stop diarrhea, says Dr. Tilghman. It also contains substances that will ease a sore throat.

Holistic veterinarians rarely use herbs alone, Dr. Tilghman adds. They often combine herbs with conventional medicines, giving your pet the best of both worlds.

Herbal remedies can be confusing at first. There are dozens of common healing herbs, and they come in many forms—fresh, dried, concentrated, and packed into capsules. Here are a few tips for making the right choice.

Pick the right form. Even when the active ingredients are the same, herbs have different effects, depending on how they are prepared and packaged, says Susan G. Wynn, D.V.M., a veterinarian in Atlanta and coeditor of *Complementary and Alternative Veterinary Medicine*.

- *Bulk herbs* can be fresh and green or dry, crumbly, or powdered. Bulk herbs are usually prepared by mixing them into food or steeping them in hot water, which releases the active compounds. The resulting teas and decoctions work quickly because they are absorbed very readily by the body.
- *Extracts and tinctures* are liquid, concentrated forms of herbs. As with herbal teas, they pass quickly through the intestinal wall and are often recommended when pets need fast relief, such as from pain. Extracts and tinctures can be mixed a drop or two at a time in a

The 15 Top Herbs

The U.S. Department of Agriculture has cataloged more than 80,000 herbs, many of which are thought to have healing powers. For the majority of health problems, however, you need only a few herbs, like these. (To be safe, talk to your vet before using them at home.)

Herb	Used to Treat
Aloe (*Aloe vera*)	Constipation, skin irritation
Calendula (*Calendula officinalis*)	Skin injuries
Chamomile (*Matricaria recutita*)	Skin irritation (topical), stomach problems, mild stress
Comfrey (*Symphytum officinale*)	Skin injuries (topical only)
Dandelion (*Taraxacum officinale*)	Water retention
Echinacea (*Echinacea angustifolia* or *Echinacea purpurea*)	Infections, inflammation

glass of water and poured on your pet's food. Or you can put them straight into your pet's mouth. Some tinctures are made by soaking herbs in alcohol, which may be dangerous—as well as unappetizing—for cats. Other tinctures are glycerin-based, which may be better for some pets. Extracts and tinctures can be quite powerful, and doses vary widely, so it is important to talk to your vet before using them.

• *Tablets and capsules* are just as effective as fresh herbs, as long as you use them before their expiration dates.

Herb	Used to Treat
Eucalyptus (*Eucalyptus globulus*)	Nasal congestion
Ginger (*Zingiber officinale*)	Nausea, motion sickness
Ginkgo (*Ginkgo biloba*)	Old age, mental dullness
Goldenseal (*Hydrastis canadensis*)	Infections, bronchial inflammation
Hawthorn (*Crataegus laevigata*)	Heart irregularities
Milk thistle (*Silybum marianum*)	Liver problems
Red clover (*Trifolium pratense*)	Bronchitis
Slippery elm (*Ulmus rubra*)	Diarrhea, constipation, coughs
Valerian (*Valeriana officinalis*)	Stress, pain, aggression

Know your supplier. Unlike drugs, which are produced and packaged with scientific precision, herbs can vary in strength from batch to batch, depending on such things as climate, soil conditions, and which fertilizers were used. The only way to be sure that you are getting the best quality is to ask your vet to recommend a reputable supplier, says Nancy Scanlan, D.V.M., a holistic veterinarian in private practice in Sherman Oaks, California.

Read the label carefully. Many herbs have similar-sounding names—for example, bitterstick, used to strengthen immunity, and bitterroot, used for asthma and breathing problems. Some manufacturers list both common and scientific names on the label, which helps prevent confusion.

Shop for freshness. Fresh and dried herbs don't last forever, says Dr. Tilghman. When buying packaged herbs, look for expiration or harvest dates on the label. When buying them in bulk form, put your nose to work. Fresh herbs should smell fresh. If they smell dry or musky, they have probably given up their essential oils and won't be as effective.

Store them carefully. Herbs quickly lose strength when they are exposed to light and heat, so be sure to store them in a cool, dark place. Some herbs react with chemicals in plastic containers, so it is better to store them in glass instead.

Flower Essences: Good Vibrations

One of the best ways to soothe nervous pets is with flower essences, says Dr. Fulp. Made from the essential (and greatly diluted) oils of wild plants, trees, and bushes, flower essences such as Bach Flower Remedies help return the body's emotional energy fields to a proper balance, she explains.

Holistic veterinarians usually use a single-flower essence to treat specific types of emotional stress. The essence mimulus is good for soothing fears. "Vervain calms nervous energy, vine helps stop aggression, and rock rose helps with terror," says Dr. Fulp. In some cases, several flower essences are combined into one remedy. The essence called Bach Rescue Remedy contains the essences impatiens, star-of-Bethlehem, cherry plum, rock rose, and clematis. "Rescue Remedy is good for any kind of stress because it helps make pets more mellow," she says.

Flower essences are harmless, and accidentally using the wrong one won't cause problems, Dr. Fulp adds. They usually work quickly, and your pet should start feeling better

Essential Essences

Holistic veterinarians often recommend flower essences for healing the emotions. Here are 12 popular ones. You can either squirt the proper amount in your pet's water bowl or put a few drops on the bridge of his nose or the pads of his paws, where they will quickly be absorbed into the body by licking.

Essence	Used to Treat
Aspen	Fear of the unknown
Beech	Intolerance
Centaury	Excessive submission
Larch	Lack of confidence
Mimulus	Fear of the known
Rescue Remedy	Mental or physical trauma
Rock rose	Terror
Star-of-Bethlehem	Shock
Vervain	Overenthusiasm
Vine	Dominance or aggression
Water violet	Aloofness
Willow	Resentment

within a few days. You can use flower essences by themselves or in combination with other therapies. In most cases, however, it is best to keep things simple, she says. "Using three or fewer at a time will usually give the best results."

Flower essences are very easy to use. "For cats, put a couple of drops in their water bowls so they sip it all day long," says Dr. Fulp. "For dogs, drip the essence directly into their mouths or put it on their noses to lick off." Veterinarians usually advise giving 1 to 3 drops a day until your pet feels better. When giving the drops directly, don't let the dropper touch your pet's skin or mouth. Otherwise, the bottle will become contaminated, she explains.

You can buy flower essences from most health food stores and some pet supply catalogs. They are usually sold near a chart or list that explains which essences are recommended for different conditions. As with most natural remedies, flower essences should be stored in glass bottles away from direct sun, microwaves, and heat.

Aromatherapy: The Power of Scents

Holistic veterinarians have discovered that certain scents act like medicines, affecting the body on a biochemical level. But rather than be absorbed from the stomach, as with pills, the fragrant scents used in aromatherapy are absorbed by the mucous membranes in the nose. The chemicals of the aromas go straight to the brain, explains Dr. Fulp.

The oils used in aromatherapy are available in health food stores and some pet supply catalogs. The oils usually come from natural sources, although synthetic (and cheaper) versions are available. As with flower essences, you can buy single oils or oil blends.

Holistic veterinarians have only recently begun working with aromatherapy, so until more is known, says Dr. Fulp, it is essential to check with your veterinarian before using aromatherapy on your own—especially because some oils, like peppermint and pennyroyal, can be dangerous or even fatal when used on pets.

Once your veterinarian has given you the proper oils, here is how to put them to work.

Dilute the oil. The essential oils used in aromatherapy are much too strong to use straight from the bottle. "Dilute the oil half-and-half with a vegetable oil like peanut oil," says Dr. Fulp. This will prevent burning if it touches the skin. Use essential oils only where your pet can't lick them off—on his ears or the back of his neck. It may be safer to use a diffuser, which vaporizes the scent into the air.

Aim for the ears. When using aromatherapy, it is important to apply the drops where the scent will reach the nose and the oils will penetrate the skin. "Massage a drop or two on the inside of the ear tip, where there is not much fur," says Dr. Fulp. "That's near the face, so the pet breathes the scent, but he can't reach it to lick it off."

Use it briefly. Unlike drugs, which may be taken for days or weeks, aromatherapy usually works very quickly. "It's almost always a short-term treatment," says Dr. Fulp. "The effects usually wear off in 4 to 6 hours, but one treatment is

How to Give Medicine

Homeopathic pills are easy to give to dogs. (Don't touch homeopathic pills with your fingers because this can reduce their effectiveness.) Grip the dog's nose with one hand and point it upward. With your other hand, pull down the lower jaw and pop the pill toward the back of the throat. Hold the mouth closed and massage the throat until you see your dog swallow. Then take a look in his mouth to be sure the pill went down.

Cats don't like taking pills and will put up a fight when you attempt it. An easier way is to use a homeopathic solution. Draw the solution into a needleless syringe or a dropper, tilt the cat's head back, and squirt the medicine into the side of the mouth.

An easy way to give liquid medication to a resistant pet is to gently pull out the back corner of the lower lip, making a pouch. With the head tilted back, pour the liquid into the pouch with the other hand. Gently hold your pet's mouth closed and briefly put your thumb over his nostrils to make him swallow.

usually enough," she says. When your pet doesn't get better right away, it is fine to use aromatherapy three times a day for 1 or 2 days. After that, call your vet, Dr. Fulp advises.

Dietary Supplements: Nutritional Cures

Even when you give your pets an all-natural, high-quality food, there is still a possibility that they aren't getting all the nutrients they really need. That is why many holistic veterinarians recommend giving dogs and cats dietary supplements—not just for maintaining overall health but also for fighting disease.

Call the Vet

Herbal remedies are often much safer than their pharmaceutical counterparts, but they still contain powerful compounds. Always check with your vet before starting herbal treatments at home, especially if your pet is taking other medications, says Allen M. Schoen, D.V.M., director of the Veterinary Institute for Therapeutic Alternatives in Sherman, Connecticut, and author of *Love, Miracles, and Animal Healing.*

Pets with heart problems, for example, are often treated with the drug digitalis. An herbal remedy for heart problems is hawthorn (*Crataegus laevigata*). When the two are given together, they can amplify each other's effects, essentially causing an overdose, says Dr. Schoen.

Another potential problem is that herbs aren't as precisely regulated as drugs. An herb from one manufacturer may be two or three times stronger than an identical herb from another manufacturer. The only way to be sure your pet is getting the right herb and the right dose is to check with your vet first.

There are diseases that have been linked to previously unrecognized deficiencies of certain nutrients, says Dr. Scanlan. "For instance, the recommended minimum amount of taurine in cat foods had to be increased in recent years because cats weren't getting enough and were developing blindness and heart disease."

Nearly all holistic veterinarians and an increasing number of mainstream vets are now recommending that dogs and cats be given vitamin C and E supplements. Both of these nutrients are powerful antioxidants that help reduce the effects of free radicals, harmful oxygen molecules that are naturally produced by the body. Supplementation with these nutrients can help slow the aging process so that pets live longer, says Dr. Scanlan.

Dietary supplements don't give fast results, she adds. Fatty-acid supplements may take a month or more before they cause noticeable improvements in skin conditions. Other supplements, like vitamin C, work slowly over a lifetime. You may not notice any difference at all in how your pet is acting or feeling. But at the cellular level, changes will be happening—changes that will help keep your pet healthy and strong for the rest of his life.

Even though many dietary supplements are quite safe, you shouldn't use them without talking to a veterinarian who is knowledgeable about nutritional therapy. For one thing, supplements may interfere with other medications that your pet may be taking. More important, every dog and cat has different needs and will require different amounts of various substances. Don't assume that the human doses listed on labels are appropriate for dogs and cats.

Water: The Liquid of Life

Holistic veterinarians believe water is one of the best "drugs" for protecting your pet's health. Water regulates his body temperature, aids in digestion, and lubricates his tissues. More important, it is constantly transporting oxygen and nutrients to cells throughout the body and carrying away the wastes.

Holistic veterinarians don't write prescriptions for water, but it is an essential part of many treatment plans. Pets with constipation are often encouraged to drink more because water lubricates the digestive tract and helps stools move smoothly, says Carin A. Smith, D.V.M., a veterinary consultant in Washington and author of *101 Training Tips for Your Cat*. Water can also flush away bacteria that cause urinary tract infections, and a high-water "diet" is often recommended for pets with urinary stones. For pets with arthritis or hip pain, using water externally—in the form of a good swim—strengthens the joints and helps prevent pain.

You can't force your pets to drink more water. What you can do is make water more appealing. Here are a few tips veterinarians recommend.

Buy bottled water. Many pets dislike the smell (and taste) of chlorine and other substances in tap water. Bottled spring water is inexpensive, and most pets prefer it to tap water.

Add a little flavoring. When you want your pet to drink more, try adding a little flavor to his water bowl by pouring in a small amount of juice from a can of clams, for example. "My dog loves the water that's left after boiling meat or chicken," Dr. Smith says.

Put gravy on the menu. One of the easiest ways to help your pets get more fluids is to moisten their dry food with a little water, says Dr. Smith. Or give them moist or canned foods, which contain a lot more water than dry kibble.

Change the bowl. Dogs and cats are extremely sensitive to odors, and plastic water bowls may develop "off" smells that discourage them from drinking more. Switching to glass or ceramic bowls will prevent odor buildups, Dr. Smith says.

PART TWO

Common Health Problems

Aging

The Signs

- Your pet sleeps more and plays less than she used to.
- She doesn't always hear you when you approach.
- She moves slowly or has trouble getting up.

We don't like to think about our pets getting old, but it is an issue that every pet owner must face. Pets typically live only a fraction of the amount of time that we do, so they age faster and need help earlier, says Albert J. Simpson, D.V.M., a holistic veterinarian in private practice in Oregon City, Oregon.

Old age isn't a disease, but it weakens many parts of the body—from the joints and muscles to the immune system—making troublesome problems much more likely to occur. "Older pets tend to get sick more easily, and it takes them longer to get well," says W. Jean Dodds, D.V.M., adjunct professor of clinical sciences at the University of Pennsylvania School of Veterinary Medicine in

Philadelphia and owner of Hemopet, a national nonprofit animal blood bank in Irvine, California.

For a long time, veterinarians focused mainly on treating the symptoms of age-related illnesses, such as using aspirin to ease arthritis. But holistic veterinarians feel that there is a better approach. Rather than treating symptoms, they look for ways to strengthen the entire body so that the pet is much less likely to get sick in the first place. "The goal is to prevent problems and not wait for trouble to develop," says Dr. Dodds.

The Solutions

Feed pets naturally. Veterinarians have found that the chemical additives and preservatives in many commercial foods, as well as the low ratio of proteins to carbohydrates in them, may speed up the aging process by causing the body to produce more waste products. The extra work involved in getting rid of the wastes can strain the kidneys, liver, and other organs, says Dr. Dodds.

Natural foods are easy to digest and produce fewer wastes than commercial foods, says Nancy Scanlan, D.V.M., a holistic veterinarian in private practice in Sherman Oaks, California. You can choose from a number of high-quality, all-natural foods, such as Innova, Solid Gold, and Wysong, which are available in some pet supply stores and through mail order, or you can make your pet's meals at home. Holistic veterinarians advise giving dogs a diet consisting of one-third meat, one-third raw vegetables, and one-third cooked carbohydrates, such as rice or potatoes. For cats, a natural-food diet should consist of one-half meat, one-quarter raw vegetables, and one-quarter cooked carbohydrates.

Decrease the servings. Older pets burn two to four times fewer calories than youthful ones. They also exercise less, so they tend to get a little tubby. The extra weight puts additional strain on muscles and joints. You have to feed them less to keep them trim and healthy, says Dr. Scanlan.

Every pet needs different amounts of food, she adds. A good way to check is with the rib test: You should be able to feel, but not see, your pet's ribs. In cats, take a look at their bellies—when there is too much sway, they need to eat a little less. "Just feed them less of the same food," says Dr. Scanlan. Start by decreasing the amount by about one-quarter. If your pet seems hungry on this amount of food, mix in a little rice, which is filling but lower in calories than her usual food.

Give a digestive aid. In nature, dogs and cats swallowed helpful digestive enzymes when they ate the internal organs of their prey. Commercial and homemade diets lack these enzymes, which means that your pets are unable to unlock the full benefits of their food. Some holistic veterinarians recommend giving older pets digestive enzymes, such as F-Biotic for cats and C-Biotic for dogs, and following the directions on the label.

Protect their joints. The cartilage in the joints is extremely tough, but it doesn't last forever. Over time, it begins to break down, causing pain and stiffness. Holistic veterinarians have found that dietary supplements containing glucosamine or a combination of glucosamine and chondroitin sulfate, like Cosequin, can help heal damaged cartilage and keep it strong in the future. You can give pets 10 milligrams of Cosequin per pound of body weight twice a day. The combination of glucosamine and chondroitin sulfate shouldn't be given to pets with liver disease or clotting disorders, says Susan G. Wynn, D.V.M., a veterinarian in Atlanta and coeditor of *Complementary and Alternative Medicine*.

Give them a massage. Older pets often tire easily, in part because their circulation isn't as efficient as it used to be. Massaging pets helps stimulate bloodflow, which nourishes tissues and washes away pain-causing lactic acid crystals, which collect in tired muscles, says Michelle Rivera, a certified massage therapist, a veterinary dental technician, and co-owner of the Healing Oasis Veterinary Hospital in Sturtevant, Wisconsin.

The best massage technique for older pets, called effleurage, involves using long, firm strokes over your pet's entire body. It keeps the muscles toned and can help prevent stiffness, says Michael W. Fox, B.V.M. (bachelor of veterinary medicine, a British equivalent of D.V.M.), Ph.D., a veterinary consultant in Washington, D.C., and author of *The Healing Touch*. Massaging your pets daily also allows you to detect problems, such as lumps beneath the skin, that you might otherwise miss, he adds.

Get them moving. Regular exercise is important for pets of all ages, and it is especially beneficial for older dogs and cats. It helps keep joints working smoothly because it literally pumps in lubricating fluids. It also strengthens the immune system and causes the body to release endorphins, natural chemicals that help relieve pain, says Dr. Dodds. Vets recommend giving pets as much exercise as they can comfortably handle. Try to get them moving by taking them on regular walks or just by playing in the house for at least 20 minutes, twice a day.

Give them extra strokes. "Many 20-year-old cats and dogs I see have spent a lifetime being handled and petted—sitting on the owner's lap, spending time with them, staying connected," says Dr. Fox. Petted and loved pets live longer, not only because they are emotionally happy but also because touch keeps the body healthy.

Gentle petting and massaging can increase circulation to muscles and decrease spasms, adds Dr. Scanlan.

Provide extra comfort. "Older pets appreciate a soft place to rest," says Dr. Simpson. You can buy pet beds—

everything from rubber mats to thickly padded foam pillows—at pet supply stores, but you don't really need anything fancier than an old blanket on the floor, he says.

Keep her warm. "Pets really appreciate having a warm light nearby," says Dr. Simpson. When using heat, however, be sure it doesn't burn the skin. Keep heat lamps several feet away from your pet's bed, says Dr. Simpson, and give your pet space to move away from the heat if she gets overheated. You can buy a heat lamp (brooder) bulb at most hardware stores or feed stores.

Raise your voice. As dogs and cats age, the tiny bones inside the ears that amplify sound tend to lose their mobility and become less sensitive. That's why your dog or cat may appear to be ignoring you or will sometimes get startled when you come up and touch her from behind. Talking more loudly will often help, says Dr. Dodds. It is also a good idea to lightly stamp your foot when you are trying to get your pet's attention but you are not in her line of sight.

Give them a boost. It is normal for dogs and cats to become a little less agile with the passing years. If your pet is accustomed to a favorite place—a window perch, for example, or a chair in the living room—you may want to put a low stool or platform underneath so that he can help himself up, says Dr. Simpson. This not only helps him get comfortable but also provides a great emotional boost since older pets may get depressed when they can't do the things that they used to.

Take her swimming. Swimming is one of the best exercises for dogs because the water supports their weight and prevents punishing strain on muscles and joints, says Dr. Fox. Swimming is great for cats, too—if they like the water. Most don't, of course, so water sports are really limited to dogs.

Allergies

The Signs

- Your pet licks or bites his feet.
- He rubs his face on the floor or against furniture.
- There is a rash on his belly.
- His nose is runny and his eyes are red.
- He keeps getting ear infections.

Cats and dogs can be allergic to many of the same things as humans, like pollen and mold. They can also be sensitive to fleas, yard chemicals, or even grass. But unlike humans, who usually sniffle and sneeze when they have allergies, pets get extremely itchy.

"Allergies mean that the immune system is being thrown off by things in the environment," says Greig Howie, D.V.M., a holistic veterinarian in private practice in Dover, Delaware. Food additives, chemicals in the air and water, and even vaccinations may cause the immune system to react to the wrong things, says Dr. Howie. That is why holistic veterinarians favor a whole-body approach—one that controls the symptoms and helps the immune system stay on track.

The Solutions

Try a simple diet. One of the best ways to calm allergies and hay fever is to give your pet a natural diet, one that doesn't contain the artificial additives found in many commercial foods, says Karen Komisar, D.V.M., a holistic veterinarian in private practice in Lynn, Massachusetts. "A natural diet often helps quiet the immune system."

The best meals for pets with allergies are those that are homemade, adds Deborah C. Mallu, D.V.M., a holistic veterinarian in private practice in Sedona, Arizona. She recommends giving dogs meals that are one-third meat (preferably raw or lightly steamed), one-third cooked grains, and one-third finely chopped vegetables. Cats need more protein than dogs. Their meals should be about 50 percent meat, 25 percent cooked grains, and 25 percent cooked vegetables.

When you don't have the time or inclination to cook from scratch, look for all-natural pet foods that don't contain chemical additives or preservatives, says Dr. Mallu. You can get natural foods from holistic veterinarians and from some pet supply or health food stores.

Calm the skin with calendula. Calendula (*Calendula officinalis*) ointment is an herbal preparation that quickly relieves itching caused by allergies, says Adriana Sagrera, D.V.M., a holistic veterinarian in private practice in New Orleans. She recommends applying a thin coat of the ointment two or three times a day to the areas your pet is scratching.

Strengthen the immune system with echinacea. Echinacea (*Echinacea purpurea* or *Echinacea angustifolia*) is a healing herb that helps the immune system work more effectively, and it is often recommended for pets with allergies, says Sandra Priest, D.V.M., a veterinarian in private practice in Knoxville, Tennessee. She recommends adding 2 to 4 drops of echinacea extract to an ounce of spring water and putting a dropperful in your pet's mouth once a day or every other day. Echinacea works best when it is given before allergies actually start—in the early spring, for example, before pollens fill the air.

Put vitamins to work. Vitamins C and E have been shown to help the body fight the inflammation that accompanies allergic reactions. You can give cats or dogs under 15 pounds 250 milligrams of vitamin C (preferably in the form of sodium ascorbate) a day during allergy season. Pets 15 pounds and over need more, usually between 500 and 1,000 milligrams a day, says Cheryl Schwartz, D.V.M., a holistic veterinarian in San Francisco and author of *Four Paws, Five Directions: A Guide to Chi-*

Call the Vet

Most pets with hay fever or allergies will be a little uncomfortable during flare-ups, but they won't have serious problems. In some cases, however, they get so itchy that they scratch themselves raw, causing sores or infections, says Karen Komisar, D.V.M., a holistic veterinarian in private practice in Lynn, Massachusetts.

When the itchiness isn't going away, or your pet has other symptoms like an eye discharge or sores or a bad odor on the skin, you need to see your vet. He may recommend allergy tests to find what your pet is allergic to. And he may give your pet medications until gentler, more natural remedies have time to work.

nese Medicine for Cats and Dogs. "If you give them too much, they get diarrhea. When that happens, lower the dose until the diarrhea goes away." Also, to avoid stomach upset, it is best to give vitamin E with food.

Vitamin E is also good for the skin, Dr. Schwartz adds. She recommends 50 international units (IU) for cats and dogs weighing less than 10 pounds. Give 200 IU to pets weighing from 10 to 40 pounds and 400 IU for dogs over 40 pounds. It should be given once a day during allergy season. As with vitamin C, give vitamin E with food, she adds.

Vitamin E increases blood pressure, adds Dr. Schwartz, so don't give it to pets with high blood pressure without first checking with your vet.

Provide some essential fats. Another way to fight skin inflammation is with essential fatty acids, found in flaxseed oil and fish oil. "In order to get a balanced anti-inflammatory effect, look for a supplement that has both omega-3 and omega-6 fatty acids," advises Dr. Priest. You can buy fatty-acid supplements made specifically for pets. Just follow the directions on the label.

Shower them with flowers. Holistic veterinarians often use flower essences to soothe itchy pets. A good combination of essences is agrimony, beech, cherry plum, crab apple, olive, and walnut, says Wanda Vockeroth, D.V.M., a holistic veterinarian in private practice in Calgary, Alberta. To prepare the mixture, put 2 or 3 drops of each essence in a 1-ounce dropper bottle filled with spring or purified water. Give your pet a dropperful of the mixture twice a day. "You can also put it in a spray bottle and spritz the itchy spots or dab some on a cloth and wipe it on," she adds.

Change their water. Chemicals in drinking water can make the immune system act a little haywire, says Anne Lampru, D.V.M., a holistic veterinarian in private practice in Tampa, Florida. "Give them distilled water for 6 to 8 weeks, which will help them slowly detoxify," she says. "Then put them on good filtered water."

Wash them with oatmeal. You can give itchy pets quick relief by washing them with an oatmeal shampoo, available in pet supply stores, says Dr. Komisar. Or, if they will put up with it, you can add some colloidal oatmeal (like Aveeno) to their bathwater and give them a soothing soak for 10 to 15 minutes.

Ease their eyes with eyebright. Pets with allergies may get weepy, itchy eyes. When they do, you may want to rinse the eyes with an herbal eyewash. Dr. Priest recommends boiling a cup of pure water and adding 2 to 4 drops of eyebright (*Euphrasia officinalis*) extract. Boil the solution for another minute, then let it cool entirely. Draw some solution into a dropper and rinse your pet's eyes once a day.

There are many conditions besides allergies that can cause red eyes, Dr. Priest adds. So if the redness doesn't go away after 2 days—or you are not sure that allergies are responsible—ask your vet to take a look. Pets that squint or paw at their eyes may be in pain, and you should call your vet right away.

Vaccinate with care. Many holistic veterinarians believe that giving pets a lot of vaccines may compromise the immune system, causing it to overreact to ordinary substances. It is worth asking your veterinarian if vaccines may be contributing to the problem and whether it is a good idea for your pet to get fewer vaccines or to get vaccinated less often.

Anal Sac Problems

The Signs
- Your pet scoots across the floor.
- He licks his bottom more than usual.
- The anal area is swollen or inflamed, or there is a discharge.

Whenever dogs or cats have a bowel movement, they release small amounts of fluid from the anal sacs—two storage areas on either side of the anus. The sacs normally empty and refill every day. When stools aren't firm enough, however, they don't exert enough pressure to empty the sacs. This causes fluid to accumulate, making the anal area itchy and sore, says Jeffrey Feinman, V.M.D., a holistic veterinarian in private practice in Fairfield County in Connecticut.

Small dogs tend to have more anal sac problems than larger breeds. Cats occasionally have blocked anal sacs, but it is generally more of a dog problem. The traditional treatment is to unblock the sacs by manually pressing out the fluid. It is an easy procedure, but the problem often comes back. That is why holistic veterinarians favor more of a whole-body—and hands-off—approach.

The Solutions

Put water to work. One of the most effective ways to relieve discomfort and help the anal sacs drain is to soak your pet's bottom in a mixture of warm water and Epsom salts (about 1 cup of salts in 2 gallons of water) for about 10 minutes, says Junia Borden Childs, D.V.M., a holistic veterinarian in private practice in Ojai, California. Doing this once or twice a day for a few days will help liquefy the fluid in the sacs so that it flows more easily. The salts can be drying, however, so it is a good idea to apply a little petroleum jelly or mineral oil after the bath, she adds.

Apply a warm compress. An easy alternative is to soak a washcloth in the Epsom salts–water mixture and hold it to your pet's rear for about 10 minutes, twice a day. "A lot of times this will open the sacs," says Dr. Childs. You can

The Healing Instinct

Dogs and cats with blocked anal sacs sometimes scoot across the floor on their bottoms. It looks as though they are giving themselves a little scratch—and they probably are. But it's also nature's way of putting extra pressure on the sacs, says Susan G. Wynn, D.V.M., a veterinarian in Atlanta and coeditor of *Complementary and Alternative Veterinary Medicine*. This can help the sacs empty, relieving the pressure and making pets feel better.

also try placing your palm over your pet's bottom and gently rocking it back and forth, without squeezing. The slight pressure often helps the sacs drain, she explains.

Try a new diet. Switching pets to a higher-quality food—one that has at least two meat sources among the first three ingredients—or giving them homemade food may help prevent blocked anal sacs, says Susan G. Wynn, D.V.M., a veterinarian in Atlanta and coeditor of *Complementary and Alternative Veterinary Medicine*.

Give your pet extra fiber. Improve your pet's diet by giving him fresh vegetables, which are high in dietary fiber. Fiber absorbs tremendous amounts of water in the intestine, which causes stools to get larger. Larger stools put more pressure on the anal sacs, helping them empty normally, says Dr. Wynn. She recommends giving cats and dogs under 15 pounds about ⅛ cup of minced vegetables, such as broccoli or carrots, each day. Pets weighing 15 to 50 pounds can have between ¼ cup and ½ cup. Dogs over 50 pounds can have as much as 2 cups of vegetables each day.

If your cat turns up his whiskers at the minced vegetables, run them through a blender—adding a little water or chicken broth—and mix them with his food.

Get those paws moving. Regular exercise strengthens the rectal and abdominal muscles so they put more pressure on the anal sacs. Healthy dogs and cats should get at least 20 minutes of exercise twice a day.

Soothe them with Silica. Silica is a homeopathic remedy that can help the anal sacs empty normally, says Allen M. Schoen, D.V.M., director of the Veterinary Institute for Therapeutic Alternatives in Sherman, Connecticut, and author of *Love, Miracles, and Animal Healing*. He recommends giving 2 or 3 drops or three to five pellets of Silica 6C twice a day for 3 days. For some pets, this is all you will need to do to relieve the discomfort.

Call the Vet

Anal sac problems usually aren't serious and clear up within a few days. But blocked anal sacs sometimes get infected. This can cause inflammation, impaction, or a painful abscess, says Susan G. Wynn, D.V.M., a veterinarian in Atlanta and coeditor of *Complementary and Alternative Veterinary Medicine*. Infections can be dangerous, so it is important to call your vet when your dog or cat is suddenly scooting a lot more than usual or the anal area looks red or swollen. Your vet may need to clean out the sacs thoroughly and possibly install a temporary "drain." Your pet may need oral antibiotics as well.

Relieve his allergies. Some anal sac problems in dogs may be related to allergies. If your dog is scratching a lot and licking his feet and he has anal sac problems, there is a good chance that the problems are related, says Dr. Wynn. If your dog can't avoid whatever he is allergic to, give him dog supplements containing omega-3 fatty acids, such as fish oil or flaxseed oil, which can help reduce itching and inflammation. Vets usually recommend giving dogs under 15 pounds 250 to 500 milligrams of fatty acids twice a day, says Dr. Wynn. Dogs between 15 and 50 pounds can have 1,000 milligrams one or two times a day. Dogs 50 pounds and over can take between 1,000 and 2,000 milligrams twice daily. Every pet reacts differently to supplements, however, so ask your vet for the correct dose.

Anemia

The Signs

- Your pet's gums are pale or white.
- The insides of her eyelids are pale, instead of pink.
- She seems weak and tired.
- Her breathing is labored, and her pulse is fast.

Anything that causes blood loss—from fleas to wounds to internal diseases—can cause anemia, a condition in which dogs and cats don't have enough red blood cells to deliver all the oxygen their bodies need. Without enough oxygen, pets get tired and weak.

Anemia is always a symptom of another, more serious problem and a warning sign that your pet needs immediate veterinary attention, says Michael W. Lemmon, D.V.M., a holistic veterinarian in Renton, Washington, and past president of the American Holistic Veterinary Medical Association.

The Solutions

Put meat on the menu. The proteins in turkey, lamb, beef, chicken, or other raw meats help dogs and cats create more red blood cells, enhancing the body's ability to transport oxygen, says Dr. Lemmon. Be sure to buy high-quality organic or free-range meats because they are less likely to contain dangerous organisms like salmonella, he adds. Or you could lightly steam the meat, says Alan M. Schoen, D.V.M., director of the Veterinary Institute for Therapeutic Alternatives in Sherman, Connecticut, and author of *Love, Miracles, and Animal Healing*. Check with your vet on the amount of meat that is appropriate for your anemic pet.

Serve a hearty stew. Boil chicken in water until it is tender, remove the bones, then add to the broth some vegetables like beets, spinach, and carrots, Dr. Lemmon suggests. Don't use onions, however, which can be dangerous for cats.

Call the Vet

Anemia is sneaky because the main cause—losing blood—isn't always obvious. It is up to you to notice the subtle signs: a sudden lack of energy, a distended abdomen, or gums that have gone from bubble-gum pink to pale or even white. If signs appear, call your vet immediately, says Jan Facinelli, D.V.M, a holistic veterinarian in private practice in Denver.

One easy test is to check your pet's stool every day, she adds. Since anemia may be caused by internal bleeding due to ulcers, for example, or more serious conditions such as cancer, stools that are much darker than usual or are black and tarry-looking are a serious warning sign, and you should call your vet right away.

Buoy the blood with the B vitamins. Bone marrow produces oxygen-carrying red blood cells. Strengthen your pet's bone marrow by supplementing her diet with a B vitamin elixir, says Jan Facinelli, D.V.M., a holistic veterinarian in private practice in Denver. Every pet needs different amounts of B vitamins, she adds, so ask your vet for the correct dose.

Add some vitamin C. This powerful nutrient helps the body soak up blood-building iron from the intestinal tract, says Junia Borden Childs, D.V.M., a holistic veterinarian in private practice in Ojai, California. Twice a day, give pets weighing less than 15 pounds 250 milligrams of vitamin C, she advises. Pets that weigh 15 pounds or more can take up to 1,000 milligrams of vitamin C a day. (Vitamin C occasionally causes diarrhea, so be prepared to cut back the amount until you find a dose that your pet can tolerate.)

Offer liquid liver. A raw-liver extract like Livaplex contains large amounts of blood-building iron and B-complex vitamins, Dr. Lemmon says. You can buy liver extracts from vets or health food stores. He recommends giving cats one-quarter to a whole capsule of Livaplex once a day. Dogs can take between one-half capsule and four capsules a day, depending on their size and overall health. Your vet will help you choose the proper dose. Don't give liver extracts without checking with your vet because they can be dangerous for dogs that have a liver disorder called copper-related hepatitis.

Give her some greens. Chlorophyll, a pigment found in plants, can help the body produce healthier blood, Dr. Lemmon says. Fresh, juiced, or powdered barley grass and wheat grass contain highly concentrated forms of chlorophyll. Mix the greens in their food. Give ¼ teaspoon to pets that weigh less than 15 pounds. Larger pets can have 1 to 2 teaspoons.

Other supplements containing chlorophyll include algae- and spirulina-based chlorophyll-complex powder. Give pets weighing up to 15 pounds ⅛ to ¼ teaspoon of the supplement once a day. Pets weighing more than 15 pounds can take up to 2 teaspoons a day.

Put herbs to work. Nettle (*Urtica dioica*), red clover (*Trifolium pratense*), and burdock root (*Arctium lappa*) are bursting with nutrients, especially iron, says herbalist Gregory L. Tilford, co-owner of Animals' Apawthecary in Conner, Montana, and author of *Edible and Medicinal Plants of the West*. The herbs can be mixed together or given separately. Once a day, give dogs a level tablespoon of the dried herbs for every 30 pounds of weight, he suggests. Add approximately ½ teaspoon to a cat's food each day. You can buy dried herbs at health food stores.

Try a homeopathic remedy. "Phosphorus is a remedy for many types of bleeding," says Dr. Facinelli. "It's one of the first homeopathic remedies to think of when you are treating anemia caused by blood loss."

She recommends giving dogs and cats three pellets of Phosphorus 30C three times a day for about 3 days. Crushing the pellets and putting them in a teaspoon of milk will make them easier to take, she adds.

Other homeopathic remedies are also recommended for anemia, depending on your pet's other symptoms. For example:

- Arsenicum album 6X may be helpful for anemic dogs and cats that are also weak, restless, or chilled, says Dr. Lemmon. Pets that weigh less than 15 pounds can take one or two pellets. Larger pets can take three to five pellets two or three times a day for up to 2 weeks.
- Sulfur 6X is often recommended when pets with anemia also have fleas or skin problems, he says. Give two to four pellets to pets weighing 15 pounds or more. Smaller pets can take one pellet two or three times a day for up to 2 weeks.

Arthritis

The Signs

- Stiffness
- Reduced mobility
- Reluctance to walk or exercise

Many dogs and cats get only a touch of arthritis and never experience anything worse than a little morning stiffness. Other pets, big dogs especially, may be seriously affected. Drugs like aspirin, cortisone, and carprofen (Rimadyl) are the conventional answers for treating arthritis, and in certain cases surgery may be needed to repair damaged joints. But even though arthritis always needs a veterinarian's care, there are many natural remedies that can relieve pain without the side effects of medications. Here is what holistic veterinarians advise.

The Solutions

Strengthen the cartilage. Veterinarians have found that two dietary supplements—glucosamine sulfate and chon-

droitin sulfate, which are available in health food stores—
can help repair damaged cartilage and increase lubrication
in the joint, reducing pain and stiffness, says Nancy
Scanlan, D.V.M, a holistic veterinarian in private practice
in Sherman Oaks, California.

A good supplement is Cosequin. Available from veterinarians, it contains both ingredients. You can give pets
10 milligrams of Cosequin per pound of body weight twice
a day. Don't give Cosequin to pets with liver problems or
clotting disorders.

Supplements containing green-lipped mussels, like
Glyco-Flex, are also helpful because they contain glu-
cosamine-like compounds, says Dr. Scanlan. Buy these
supplements from vets and some pet supply catalogs.
Follow the dosage directions on the label.

Give Mobility. Specialists in traditional Chinese medicine have found that an herbal combination called Mobility 2 can help pets with arthritis move more easily, says

The Healing Instinct

After resting, pets launch into a fairly vigorous
stretching routine, explains Albert J. Simpson, D.V.M.,
a holistic veterinarian in private practice in Oregon
City, Oregon. First, they arch their backs. Then they bow
their backs, putting their heads down and their tails in
the air. They finish up by taking a few steps forward
while stretching each hind leg behind them. This is nature's way of keeping joints limber and helping prevent
painful problems such as arthritis.

While dogs do a little bit of stretching, cats do a lot
more—and it pays off. "Cats don't get a lot of joint
problems," says Dr. Simpson.

Dr. Scanlan. Available from veterinarians, the usual dose is one-half tablet twice a day for cats and dogs weighing less than 15 pounds and one to two tablets twice a day for larger pets.

Flex the spine. You can use a touch technique called motion palpation to limber up the back and relieve general stiffness and discomfort, says Albert J. Simpson, D.V.M., a holistic veterinarian in private practice in Oregon City, Oregon. Beginning at the shoulders and working backward to the hips, simultaneously press with your thumb and forefinger in the depressions on either side of the spine between pairs of vertebrae. Press for 2 to 3 seconds, release, then move to the next spot, he advises. You can repeat the massage once a day until your pet feels better, he says.

Rub away the pain. A daily massage can get blood flowing into the muscles and quickly relax painful tightness, says Patricia Whalen-Shaw, a registered massage therapist and owner of Optissage, an animal massage school in Circleville, Ohio.

She recommends starting with a technique called effleurage, in which you use slow, firm strokes, beginning at the head and working back to the tail. After your pet is feeling warm and relaxed, hold your fingertips together and rub firm circles into the muscles. Concentrate on the muscles on either side of the spine, around the hips, and on the shoulders—wherever your pet seems to be hurting, Whalen-Shaw says. You can continue the massage for 15 minutes to an hour, once a day.

Give daily vitamins. Vitamin C and E supplements can reduce inflammation in the joints and protect the cartilage. Dr. Simpson recommends giving cats and dogs weighing less than 15 pounds about 10 international units (IU) of vitamin E a day. Pets 15 to 50 pounds can take 20 IU, and larger dogs can take 30 IU. For vitamin C, give about ¼ teaspoon of 1,000-milligram vitamin C powder to dogs over 50 pounds, ⅛ teaspoon of 500-milligram powder to dogs 15 to 50 pounds, and just a sprinkling (about 250 milligrams) of 500-milligram powder to smaller pets. Vitamin C can cause diarrhea, so you may have to reduce the dose until you find an amount your pet will tolerate. Dr. Simpson recommends using ester vitamin C because it is less likely to cause diarrhea. "Just sprinkle it once a day on their food," he says.

Keep them moving. Even gentle exercise may be uncomfortable at first, but the joints and muscles will quickly relax and loosen, says Dr. Simpson. It is a good idea to begin with about 5 minutes of gentle exercise twice a day, working up to 20 minutes twice a day as soon as your pet can handle it.

Stop the swelling. "An herb called boswellia (*Boswellia serrata*) naturally fights joint inflammation," says Dr. Simpson. Veterinarians usually recommend 150 to 200 milligrams twice a day. Every pet is different, however, so ask your vet for the correct dose.

Lead them to water. For dogs especially, swimming is one of the best exercises because the water supports the body and takes the strain off tender joints. Some dogs take to water naturally, but others need a little coaxing. Once you get them in, they will often stick around as they discover that the water helps soothe their pain, says Kathy Kern, a registered veterinary technician and owner of Animal Fitness Center at Almaden Valley Animal Hospital in San Jose, California.

Dogs are natural swimmers, but it is important to stay nearby to bail them out if they need some help, she says. While large dogs need 3 to 4 feet of water for swimming, smaller pets can make do in a shallow pool or even a bathtub. "I recommend 88° to 92°F water for the best results," Kern says. Let your dog swim for about 10 minutes at first. You want him to be breathing hard when he is done, but not gasping. Afterward, towel him dry and finish up with a blow-dryer, set on low and held at least 6 inches from the fur.

Add some spice to his life. The scent of essential oil of ginger (*Zingiber officinale*) can help relieve inflammation in the joints, says Teresa Fulp, D.V.M., a holistic veterinarian in private practice in Springfield, Virginia. Dilute the oil half-and-half with peanut oil, then massage it on the inside tip of your dog's ear, she advises.

Back Problems

The Signs

- Your pet hunches her shoulders, neck, or back.
- She has trouble moving.
- She cries when you pet her or pick her up.
- She limps, or her hind legs wobble when she walks.

Dogs and cats don't walk upright, so their backs do a lot less bending and twisting than ours. But even small problems like a pulled muscle or a spot of arthritis can cause a lot of pain and stiffness. Back pain is particularly common in long-bodied dogs, such as dachshunds, because their stretched-out shapes provide relatively little support for the spine, leaving them prone to injuries like herniated disks.

Traditional treatments include drugs, weeks of confinement and rest, and sometimes surgery. Except in the most serious cases, natural remedies like gentle exercise and dietary supplements relieve the pain and, in some cases, slow the progression of the underlying problem, says Susan G. Wynn, D.V.M., a veterinarian in Atlanta and coeditor of *Complementary and Alternative Veterinary Medicine*.

The Solutions

Put pressure to work. When your pet is suddenly stiff and sore, feel the muscles along either side of the spine. If you discover a hard little muscle "knot"—the telltale sign of a muscle spasm—press directly on the spot with your thumb or finger, says Dr. Wynn. Maintain the pressure for 10 seconds to 2 minutes. "You may be able to feel the knot suddenly relax," she says. Then move farther along the spine, pressing muscle spasms as you go. Muscle spasms are tender, and your pet won't like the pressure, but it is one way to stop the pain.

Ease it with ice. Back problems are often accompanied by inflammation, which puts pressure on nearby muscles and nerves. To relieve temporary pain and inflammation, apply cold to the area. You can freeze water in a paper cup, then peel away the paper to use the "ice stick" on areas that feel hot to the touch, says Randy Caviness, D.V.M., clinical instructor of small animal acupuncture at Tufts University School of Veterinary Medicine in North Grafton, Massachusetts, and a holistic veterinarian in private practice in Concord. Apply the cold for 15 to 20 minutes or until your pet makes it clear she has had enough. Repeat the treatment two or three times a day for a few days until the inflammation goes away, he advises. You will know that your pet is feeling better when she is less sensitive to touch and moves more easily.

Add a little heat. When your pet has long-term back pain that isn't accompanied by swelling, you may want to

Call the Vet

Any back problem is potentially serious. Don't take chances if the symptoms came on suddenly. Serious back problems that cause paralysis of the hind legs are an emergency, and you need to get your pet to the vet right away.

apply warmth to the area. This loosens muscles, relieving painful stiffness, says Dr. Caviness. He recommends wrapping a hot-water bottle in a towel and holding it on your pet's back for about 20 minutes, three times a day, for 2 to 3 days.

Protect the joints. Glucosamine, a supplement available in health food stores, can help heal connective tissues between the vertebrae, says Albert J. Simpson, D.V.M., a holistic veterinarian in private practice in Oregon City, Oregon. He recommends giving cats 3 to 4 milligrams of glucosamine per pound of body weight once a day. Dogs under 15 pounds can take 5 milligrams per pound, and larger dogs can take up to 15 milligrams per pound, he says.

Some veterinarians recommend giving Cosequin, a combination of glucosamine and chondroitin sulfate, which can help repair damaged cartilage. You can give pets 10 milligrams of it per pound of body weight twice daily, says Dr. Wynn. Glucosamine is safe, but when combined with chondroitin, it may cause bleeding problems. Cosequin is available only through your veterinarian and should not be used in pets that have liver problems or clotting disorders.

Walk it off. Veterinarians have traditionally recommended that dogs and cats with back problems be kept virtually immobile until they start feeling better. Holistic veterinarians feel that it is better to keep them moving, at least in a gentle way. For pets with chronic back problems, gentle, sustained exercise can help muscles stabilize the spine, Dr. Wynn says. (For pets with neck problems, use a harness instead of a collar when taking walks.) But keep in mind that pushing too hard before an injury is healed will slow recovery rather than speed it along.

Start with 5 minutes of gentle walking three to five times a week, says Dr. Wynn. As your pet gets better, gradually increase the duration of the walks from 20 to 60 minutes a day. Be sure to check with your vet before starting an exercise program, she adds. It may not be good for pets with serious injuries.

Watch her weight. Overweight pets are more likely to have back problems because of the extra pressure on the spine. Helping them lose a few pounds can relieve or even eliminate some back problems, says Nancy Scanlan, D.V.M., a holistic veterinarian in private practice in Sherman Oaks, California. To check your pet's weight, feel her sides. If you can feel the ribs, but they aren't clearly visible, she is probably in good shape. If she seems a little heavy, cut back on her food a bit or ask your vet to recommend a safe weight-loss plan.

Head for the water. Swimming is almost the perfect exercise for dogs with back problems because the water supports their weight and reduces stress on the spine. It also gets the joints moving, which loosens tight muscles and eases pain and stiffness, says Kathy Kern, a registered veterinary technician and owner of Animal Fitness Center at Almaden Valley Animal Hospital in San Jose, California.

Bad Breath

The Signs
- Your pet's breath has taken a turn for the worse recently.
- His breath smells like ammonia or urine, or it is unusually sweet.

Even though occasional bad breath is normal, foul odors that don't go away usually mean that something is wrong, either in the mouth itself or somewhere else in the body, says Kimberly Henneman, D.V.M., a holistic veterinarian in private practice in Utah. Brushing your pet's teeth won't hurt and may in fact solve the problem, but holistic veterinarians usually take a broader view.

In most cases, you can improve your pet's breath with a combination of basic hygiene and changes in his diet, along with a variety of all-natural remedies that attack the problem from the inside out. Here are a few tips you may want to try.

The Solutions

Give them some leafy greens. Fresh alfalfa and parsley contain compounds such as chlorophyll that can aid digestion and sweeten the breath, says Dr. Henneman. Finely chop parsley or alfalfa sprouts and sprinkle ½ to 1 teaspoon on your pet's food every day. Or use dried parsley. Soak 1 tablespoon in a cup of hot filtered water and let cool to room temperature. Strain and add to your pet's food. Pets under 15 pounds can take ½ to 1 teaspoon of the tea. Give 1 teaspoon to 1 tablespoon to pets weighing 15 to 50 pounds and 1 to 3 tablespoons to larger dogs.

Remove the plaque. Brushing your pet's teeth will help remove plaque. Brushing twice a day is ideal, says Anthony Shipp, D.V.M., a veterinarian in private practice in Beverly Hills, California. Twice a week, however, is okay.

Use a toothbrush made especially for dogs and cats, or rub the outer surfaces of their teeth with a small piece of gauze coated with a dab of pet toothpaste, such as Doctors Foster and Smith All Natural Toothpaste. Don't use human toothpastes because they may contain ingredients that can cause stomach upset in pets, says Wendy Beers, D.V.M., a veterinarian in private practice in Albany, California. This is especially important if your pet is currently being treated with homeopathy.

Give them dry food. Moist foods stick to the teeth, which encourages foul-smelling bacteria to proliferate. "Switching to dry food may help to improve mouth odor," says Lisa Freeman, D.V.M., Ph.D., assistant professor and clinical nutritionist at Tufts University School of Veterinary Medicine in North Grafton, Massachusetts. Cats may need both wet and dry food because they don't always drink a lot of water and can use the extra fluids they get from moist foods.

Take advantage of nature's toothbrush. Raw carrots act like natural tooth scrapers, says Cheryl Schwartz, D.V.M., a holistic veterinarian in San Francisco and author of *Four Paws, Five Directions: A Guide to Chinese Medicine for Cats and Dogs*. If your pet is reluctant to eat carrots, try freezing them first to make them more tempting.

Settle the stomach. Bad breath is often caused by indigestion. Ginger (*Zingiber officinale*) helps calm an upset stomach, says Susan G. Wynn, D.V.M., a veterinarian in Atlanta and coeditor of *Complementary and Alternative Medicine*. Add 1 tablespoon of fresh sliced ginger to a cup of hot filtered water and let cool. Strain and give pets under 15 pounds ½ to one teaspoon of the tea, using a dropper or needleless syringe, she says. Give 1 teaspoon to 1 tablespoon to pets weighing 15 to 50 pounds and 1 to 3 tablespoons to larger dogs.

Care for the gums. Smelly breath can come from a gum infection. Heal the gums with the supplement coenzyme Q_{10}, says Ihor Basko, D.V.M., a holistic veterinarian in private practice in Honolulu and Kilauea, Hawaii. He recommends giving pets weighing up to 20 pounds 10 milligrams of coenzyme Q_{10} a day. Pets 21 to 50 pounds can take up to 30 milligrams once a day, and larger dogs can take 30 milligrams twice a day.

Shed some light on the problem. Suddenly pungent breath may be caused by something that is stuck in the mouth. Place one hand over the muzzle and gently open the lower jaw with your other hand. Pets may bite when they are in pain, so be cautious. Use a flashlight to take a look inside. If you see something stuck between the teeth or under the gum, have it removed by your vet.

Bladder-Control Problems

The Signs
- Your pet dribbles urine while she sleeps.
- Her bedding or back legs are wet.
- She has started having accidents in the house.

Even well-trained dogs may lose control occasionally or for prolonged periods of time. Spayed female dogs are the ones most likely to have problems with bladder control because they produce so little estrogen, a hormone that gives tension to the urinary sphincter (the muscle that controls urination), says George Carley, D.V.M., a holistic veterinarian in private practice in Tulsa, Oklahoma. Urinary tract infections, which are readily treated with antibiotics, can also cause a loss of control. In addition, older pets, both males and females, sometimes lose control. Cats almost never have bladder-control problems, he adds.

Conventional veterinarians sometimes give dogs a form of synthetic estrogen called diethylstilbestrol or an over-the-counter "diet" medication that strengthens and tightens the urinary sphincter. Nature has provided many sources of estrogen, however, so it isn't always necessary to resort to drugs, says Dr. Carley. Here are some natural remedies you may want to try.

The Solutions

Rebalance the body. Some holistic vets treat bladder-control problems with a homeopathic combination called Urinary Incontinence. It helps change your dog's hormonal balance so the bladder and urinary sphincter work more efficiently. Give half a dropperful of the remedy twice a day until things start to improve, recommends Joanne Stefanatos, D.V.M., a holistic veterinarian in private practice in Las Vegas.

Replace estrogen with glandular supplements. Supplements containing extracts from the ovaries and the adrenal, thyroid, and pituitary glands may help. Called raw-gland concentrates or multiple-glandular dietary supplements, these products help the body produce more natural estrogen, says Dr. Carley.

Holistic veterinarians sometimes use a product called Symplex F, available from veterinarians only, which contains all the necessary extracts. Or you can use a glandular supplement designed for humans, such as Solaray, available in health food stores, says Anne Lampru, D.V.M., a holistic veterinarian in private practice in Tampa, Florida. She recommends giving dogs weighing under 15 pounds one-quarter of the human dose. Dogs 15 to 50 pounds can take one-third of the human dose, and larger dogs can take one-half. Most dogs will need to take the supplements for the rest of their lives, she adds.

Strengthen the nerves with massage. Back and spinal disk injuries sometimes put pressure on the nerves that control urination, resulting in incontinence, says Susan G. Wynn, a veterinarian in Atlanta and coeditor of *Complementary and Alternative Veterinary Medicine*. You can use a technique called motion palpation to flex the spine and reduce pressure on the nerves.

Hold your thumb and index finger together and find the dip between two vertebrae on either side of your pet's backbone. Gently press straight down for 1 to 2 seconds, then release. (Some pets are sensitive to the pressure, so you may want to press with the flat of your hand.) Starting at the shoulders and going to the hips, press between each pair of vertebrae, using just enough pressure to slightly move the spine. Because motion palpation helps keep the spine flexible, it can help prevent as well as treat incontinence, says Dr. Wynn.

Keep the mind sharp. Older dogs sometimes forget that they are supposed to wait until they get outside. Vitamins A, C, and E seem to help, says Dr. Wynn. She recommends a supplement called Cell-Advance, available from veterinarians; follow the directions on the label.

Digestive enzymes such as Prozyme and FloraZyme, available in pet supply stores, may also help the intestines absorb nutrients more efficiently, which can play a role in keeping the mind sharp, explains Dr. Carley. Follow the label directions. (An alternative is yogurt containing active cultures. Pets under 15 pounds can have a few teaspoons at every meal, and larger pets can have a few tablespoons.)

Egg yolks also act as natural digestion enzymes, says Roger L. DeHaan, D.V.M., a holistic veterinarian in private practice in Frazee, Minnesota. Pets under 50 pounds can have one yolk a week, and larger pets can have two, he explains.

Bloat

The Signs

- Your dog's belly is swollen.
- He tries to vomit, but nothing comes up.
- He drools heavily.

Humans who eat too much sometimes get a gassy, bloated feeling. It is uncomfortable and sometimes embarrassing, but it is not a serious problem. In dogs, however, bloat (also called gastric dilation) can be serious or even life-threatening.

Bloat occurs when air and gases accumulate in the stomach, causing it to swell like a balloon. When bloat comes on suddenly, the stomach may swell so much that it twists within the abdominal cavity, possibly cutting off its supply of blood, explains Maria Chelaru-Williams, D.V.M., a veterinarian in private practice in Boulder, Colorado. Cats rarely get bloat, she adds. It is most common in large, deep-chested dogs like German shepherds and standard poodles.

Bloat is always an emergency, so get your pet to the vet as quickly as possible for treatment. But prevention is quite simple. Here is what veterinarians advise.

The Solutions

Feed him yogurt. Your dog's digestive tract contains bacteria that help food digest properly. When there aren't enough of these bacteria, bloat-causing gas may accumulate, says Sandra Priest, D.V.M., a holistic veterinarian in private practice in Knoxville, Tennessee. To prevent gas, "I usually suggest plain yogurt," she says. Dogs over 15 pounds can have a teaspoonful of live-culture yogurt once a day, while smaller dogs can have between ¼ and ½ teaspoon.

Add some enzymes. Digestive enzymes, available at pet supply stores, improve digestion, says Dr. Priest. Follow the directions on the label.

Divide the meals. Dogs that gobble their food are more likely to get bloat than those that eat more slowly and more often, says Monique Maniet, D.V.M., a holistic veterinarian in private practice in Bethesda, Maryland. "Try feeding your pet twice a day, and if he is still having problems, increase the frequency to three times a day," she suggests.

Let him eat in peace. Dogs often bolt their food because they are afraid other pets might get to it first. This type of anxious eating can cause gas, says Cheryl Schwartz, D.V.M., a holistic veterinarian in San Francisco and author of *Four Paws, Five Directions: A Guide to Chinese Medicine for Cats and Dogs.* "Give him his own space to eat in," she suggests.

Switch to moist food. Veterinarians often recommend moist or semimoist food instead of dry kibble. Dry dog food absorbs tremendous amounts of water in the stomach, causing it to suddenly swell, explains Dr. Maniet.

Call the Vet

Bloat can occur very quickly, sometimes causing the stomach to expand and twist (a condition called volvulus) in an hour or less. That's why it is critical to know the warning signs of bloat before it goes too far.

Dogs with sudden bloat will get a hard, swollen abdomen, which, if you tap it with your finger, will thump like a drum. They will also be uncomfortable and will arch their backs, lick their lips, drool heavily, and try to swallow. They will try to vomit, although nothing will come out. These symptoms mean that your dog is seriously ill, and you need to get him to your veterinarian or an emergency clinic immediately.

An alternative is to moisten dry food with water and let it stand for a few minutes. This allows the food to expand before it goes into your pet's stomach.

Start cooking at home. Dogs given a healthful, home-made diet are less likely to bloat, says Susan G. Wynn, D.V.M., a veterinarian in Atlanta and coeditor of *Complementary and Alternative Veterinary Medicine*.

Calm the tummy with chamomile. This healing herb may help prevent bloat, says Dr. Schwartz. "Just brew a cup of chamomile tea and cool it to room temperature," she suggests. Give dogs under 15 pounds ½ teaspoon of chamomile tea a day. Dogs 15 pounds and over can have 1 tablespoon a day. You can mix the tea in their food or put it in their mouths before meals with a needleless syringe.

Work it out. Food can ferment in sluggish intestines, causing gas to accumulate, says Dr. Priest. Counteract that by taking your dog for a brisk walk at least once a day.

Just be sure to exercise him before—not after—he eats because vigorous exercise after meals may actually cause bloat, adds Dr. Chelaru-Williams. "Wait at least 2 hours after meals before exercising," she advises.

Nix it with Nux. The homeopathic remedy Nux vomica can help reverse the buildup of gas right away, says Adriana Sagrera, D.V.M., a holistic veterinarian in private practice in New Orleans. She recommends two pellets of a 30C dose every half-hour or two pellets of a 6C dose every 15 minutes when your dog seems to be bloating.

Car Sickness

The Signs
- Your pet vomits during or shortly after a ride.
- He pants excessively or drools in the car.
- He has trouble relaxing when riding.

While most dogs and some cats learn to enjoy car rides, others work themselves into a frenzy, literally making themselves sick. Emotional stress aside, riding in a car can stimulate the vomiting center in the brain, with predictable results.

Traditional vets often recommend behavior modification techniques, along with medications, to prevent car sickness. Veterinarians who specialize in natural healing are more inclined to favor an all-natural plan customized to the individual pet. And they recommend these approaches.

The Solutions
Give your car good energy. If your pet has bad associations with the car, make it a fun place to be, says Joanne

Hibbs, D.V.M., a veterinarian in private practice in Powell, Tennessee. Stock the car with your pet's favorite chew toys, blankets, and treats. "Don't even go anywhere at first," she adds. "Just let her explore, pet her, and make her feel good." If you do this often enough, she will learn that the car is a place where good things happen, and she will be less likely to get sick in the future.

Give a little ginger. This traditional remedy works very well for nausea. "I use the capsules that are sold in health food stores," says John Limehouse, D.V.M., a holistic veterinarian in private practice in Toluca Lake, California. Dogs 15 pounds and over can take 500 milligrams of ginger (*Zingiber officinale*), while smaller pets can take half that amount or less. The easiest way to give ginger is to open a capsule and sprinkle the contents on a tablespoon of baby food. Give it about 20 minutes before going for a drive.

Cats usually won't eat ginger, so you may want to make a tea, says Susan G. Wynn, D.V.M., a veterinarian in Atlanta and coeditor of *Complementary and Alternative Veterinary Medicine*. Add 1 teaspoon of fresh grated ginger to a cup of hot water. Let it cool, strain it, and add a drop of honey. Squirt a half to a whole dropperful of the tea into the corner of your cat's mouth.

Try some Chinese herbs. A traditional Chinese remedy called Pill Curing helps treat and prevent nausea, says Dr. Limehouse. You can put these tiny pills directly on your pet's tongue, where they will dissolve. About 20 minutes before a car trip, give one vial of pills to dogs over 50 pounds. Pets 15 to 50 pounds can take 10 to 15 pills, and smaller pets can take 10 pills. For very small pets or for pets that won't swallow the pills, dilute them first in a tablespoon of lukewarm water and use a dropper to squirt it in their mouths.

Tame the tummy with Tabacum. Homeopathic Tabacum helps quell all kinds of nausea, says Arthur Young, D.V.M., a holistic veterinarian in private practice in Stuart, Florida. He suggests putting a few pellets of Tabacum 30C on your pet's tongue up to 2 hours before traveling.

Ease their emotions. An effective way to reduce emotional stress—and the nausea that often accompanies it—is to use flower essences. Dr. Young recommends putting 3 drops of premixed scleranthus into your pet's mouth. This essence balances the inner ear.

Train the brain. Even though nausea is caused by physical signals between the inner ear and brain, there are ways to "train" pets to be less sensitive, says Dr. Hibbs. She recommends taking your pet for a short drive once a week—just around the block is plenty. After three or four rides, double the distance and go out two or three times a week. Keep taking her for longer and longer drives, with some downtime in between. By gradually getting your pet used to the motion, her brain will "learn" that the sensations she feels are harmless, and the car sickness should gradually fade, she says.

Put out the lights. A simple way to prevent car sickness in cats is to put them in a small crate or box and cover it with a towel to block out the light, says Dr. Hibbs. Cats feel more secure in the dark, she explains. Don't try this in hot weather, however, because they could overheat, she says.

Cat Flu

The Signs
- Your cat sneezes a lot.
- He has a stuffy or runny nose.
- He has an eye discharge or sores on the eye, tongue, or mouth.
- He refuses to eat.

You're not the only one who can get the flu. Your cat can get a similar type of upper respiratory infection, known as cat flu.

"Vaccinations can protect cats against the most common causes of cat flu, but none are 100 percent effective," says Alice Wolf, D.V.M., professor of medicine at Texas A&M University College of Veterinary Medicine in College Station. Also, repeated vaccinations can affect the immune system, causing it to work abnormally. Holistic vets feel that it's best to supplement vaccinations with strengthening your cat's immune system naturally so he doesn't get sick in first place.

Even if he does get cat flu, the illness usually isn't serious and will go away on its own within a week, Dr. Wolf adds. To keep your cat more comfortable in the meantime—and to strengthen his defenses so that he is better protected—here are some natural treatments you may want to try.

The Solutions

Help him breathe with aromatherapy. It is hard for cats to breathe when they are congested. An effective way to break up mucus and open the airways is with a combination of essential oils called Immupower, says Teresa Fulp, D.V.M., a holistic veterinarian in private practice in Springfield, Virginia. "Dilute the oil half-and-half with peanut or pure vegetable oil and rub a little bit on the ear tip every 4 to 6 hours." Doing this once a day while your cat is sick will keep him breathing easily, says Dr. Fulp. Immupower is too concentrated to use straight and should always be diluted first.

Cook a healing meal. Chicken soup seasoned with garlic can relieve congestion and strengthen the immune system, says Pat Zook, D.V.M., a holistic veterinarian in private practice in Stone Mountain, Georgia. Homemade soup is best, although canned soup seasoned with garlic may also help. Since cats with cat flu often lose their appetites, the soup can be especially helpful because most cats relish warm broth and will eat it with gusto. You can give 4 to 8 ounces of soup a day for 2 to 3 days.

Don't overdo the garlic, Dr. Zook adds. It can cause a type of anemia. For most cats, 1/8 teaspoon a day for up to a couple of weeks is plenty. "If you are smelling garlic on his breath, you are probably getting enough in there." Also, don't use onions in the soup; they can be dangerous for cats.

Give a tomato chaser. "Tomato juice helps open the lungs, and some cats really like it," says Dr. Zook. She recommends a few tablespoons of warm tomato juice a day.

Give a vitamin boost. Research has shown that vitamin C may shorten the duration of upper respiratory viral infections and make the symptoms less severe. Dr. Zook recommends adding 125 to 250 milligrams of vitamin C powder to your cat's food every day until he is feeling better. Or you can mix the vitamin C in tomato juice or cool chicken soup, draw it up in a needleless syringe, and squirt it directly in your cat's mouth.

Clear the discharge. A homeopathic remedy called Kali bichromicum can help relieve congestion when there is a sticky, yellow nasal discharge, says Dr. Zook. Dissolve one or two 6X or 15X tablets in water, then use your fingertip to rub the solution on your cat's gums. You can do this every few hours for up to 2 days, she says.

Keep him clean. Cat flu often causes a heavy nasal discharge that blocks the nostrils and may irritate the eyes, says Carin A. Smith, D.V.M., a veterinary consultant in the state of Washington and author of *101 Training Tips for Your Cat*. She recommends using a soft, damp cloth to remove the discharge at least once a day. You may have to hold the cloth on the discharge for a while until it softens and easily wipes away.

Keep an eye on fever. It's normal for cats to run a fever when they have cat flu (normal cat temperature is 101° to 102.5°F). "A fever means the body's immune system is working overtime," says Donna M. Starita, D.V.M., a holistic veterinarian in private practice in Boring, Oregon.

You will need to call your vet, however, if the fever is 103.5° or higher or when a lower-grade fever lasts more than a day or two.

Fill the airways with humidity. Moist heat is one of the best ways to open up clogged noses and airways, says Dr. Smith. She recommends putting a humidifier near where your cat sleeps. To quickly fill his lungs with moisture, you can also take your cat with you into the bathroom when you bathe or shower, she says.

Keep him eating. When cats get congested, they lose their sense of smell, and this can cause them to stop eating, says Dr. Wolf. Until your cat's better, she says, give him foods that are smellier than usual, such as meat baby food, or add the water from canned tuna or clams.

Claw Problems

The Signs
- Your pet's paws click when she walks.
- Her nails are split and cracked.
- Her toes are swollen, or there is crusty skin around the nails.

Evolution gave dogs strong, blunt toenails for digging, while cats have razor-sharp claws for hunting and climbing trees. Life on the wild side naturally kept claws trim. But modern pets need their nails trimmed because long claws and nails tend to catch on rough surfaces and tear. Or the nails curl back and grow into the skin.

Trimming doesn't necessarily keep the nails healthy, however. Cats with weakened immune systems, for example, often get nail-bed infections, and mineral deficiencies can cause nails to crack, says George Carley, D.V.M., a holistic veterinarian in private practice in Tulsa,

Oklahoma. But there is a lot you can do to keep nails and claws healthy, say veterinarians.

The Solutions

Treat damaged nails with an herbal rinse. The herb calendula (*Calendula officinalis*), available as a tincture, reduces inflammation and helps damaged nails heal. You can even use it as a styptic to stop bleeding, says Donna M. Starita, D.V.M., a holistic veterinarian in private practice in Boring, Oregon.

You can use calendula by itself or mix it with St. John's wort (*Hypericum perforatum*). The advantage of using the combination treatment is that St. John's wort reduces swelling and helps kill bacteria and fungi. Add a teaspoon of each tincture to ¼ cup of water and rinse your pet's nails and nail beds in the solution once a day, she advises.

Keep claws healthy with fatty acids. Unhealthy nails are often caused by a dietary deficiency. Giving your pet fatty-acid supplements will help reduce inflammation and boost the immune system, says Dr. Starita. She recommends giving dogs and cats with nail problems Eskimo Oil, a supplement available from veterinarians. Cats can take ⅛ teaspoon of Eskimo Oil twice a day. Dogs 50 pounds or less can have ¼ teaspoon, and larger dogs can take ½ teaspoon twice a day.

Increase body moisture with rehmannia root. In older pets especially, the body may eliminate too much water, leading to dry, cracked nails. A Chinese herb known as rehmannia root helps the body conserve fluid by strengthening the kidneys, says Dr. Carley. He recommends a product called Six Flavor Tea Pills. It is available in some health food stores and catalogs and from veterinarians. Give pets under 15 pounds ½ to 1 tablet twice a day, he advises. Pets that weigh 15 to 50 pounds can take 1 to 2 tablets twice a day, and larger dogs can take as many as 3 tablets three times a day.

Keep them clipped. One of the best ways to prevent cracked or splintered nails is to give dogs and cats regular pedicures, says Dr. Starita. Most cats are ready for a trim every week. For dogs, every 2 to 3 weeks is plenty. Most pets hate having their nails trimmed, so you may want to spread it out over several days, doing a nail or two at a time.

Give them extra zinc. Dogs and cats that don't get enough zinc sometimes develop weak nails. You can give pets 20 milligrams of zinc gluconate for every 10 pounds of body weight once a day for 2 to 4 weeks, says Susan G. Wynn, D.V.M., a veterinarian in Atlanta and coeditor of *Complementary and Alternative Veterinary Medicine*.

Constipation

The Signs

- Your pet hasn't had a bowel movement in 48 hours.
- He cries or strains when passing stools.
- The stools are hard and dry.

Occasional constipation is fairly common and doesn't cause problems. When it lasts more than a day, however, stools in the intestine get dry and even harder to pass. Eventually, the lining of the bowel can become inflamed.

Laxatives for pets relieve constipation, but holistic veterinarians don't like using them too much because they do nothing to correct the underlying problem. A better approach, they say, is to find a long-term, natural solution for the problem that is causing constipation in the first place. Here is what they advise.

The Solutions

Ease discomfort with lavender. Holistic veterinarians recommend aromatherapy for many types of stress, including stress in the intestines. For pets with constipation, lavender essential oil is a good choice, says Donna M. Starita, D.V.M., a holistic veterinarian in private practice in Boring, Oregon. Dab a little bit of the oil, diluted half-and-half with peanut oil, where your pet can't lick it off—on his ears, for example, or the back of his neck. The oil stays active for 4 to 6 hours, so repeat the treatment several times a day until the constipation is relieved, she says.

Lubricate his insides. To help stools travel more easily through the intestine when your pet is constipated, add between ½ and 1 teaspoon of olive or safflower oil to his food, says Joanne Stefanatos, D.V.M., a holistic veterinarian in private practice in Las Vegas.

Calm the gut with Nux vomica. This homeopathic remedy helps correct energy imbalances in the intestine that can lead to constipation, says Kathleen Carson, D.V.M., a holistic veterinarian in private practice in Hermosa Beach, California. She recommends using Nux vomica liquid of 6C strength. Dilute 20 drops in an ounce of spring water and give one-half dropperful three times a day until the constipation goes away.

Firm the stools with fiber. Dietary fiber is one of the best remedies for constipation because it absorbs a tremendous amount of water in the intestine. It makes stools larger and stimulates the colon to work more efficiently. Dr. Stefanatos suggests adding psyllium husks or flaxseeds, both of which are very high in fiber, to your pet's food.

Oat bran and unflavored Metamucil are also good fiber choices, says H. Ellen Whiteley, D.V.M., a veterinary consultant in Guadalupita, New Mexico, and consultant for *The Country Vet's Home Remedies for Cats*. Whichever source of fiber you use, plan on giving about ½ teaspoon per meal to cats and to dogs weighing less than 15 pounds. Dogs 15 to 50 pounds can have a teaspoon, and dogs over 50 pounds can have a tablespoon.

Keep him comfortable with slippery elm. A healing herb that is often used for throat problems, slippery elm (*Ulmus rubra*) works for intestinal discomfort as well. "The constant straining of constipation can irritate the gut, and slippery elm bark really helps," says Dr. Carson. She recommends diluting 20 drops of slippery elm tincture in an ounce of spring water and giving your pet a dropperful three or four times a day. It is best to use tinctures that are alcohol-free because alcohol may harm cats.

Keep them active. Regular exercise strengthens the abdominal muscles, making them better able to push stools out of the body, says Dr. Whiteley. Most dogs and cats need a minimum of 20 to 30 minutes of exercise twice a day, although older pets or those with physical problems may need less, she says.

Flush them with fluids. Dogs and cats may get constipated when there isn't enough water in the intestines to help stools move smoothly. "Cats are notorious for not drinking much water," says Dr. Whiteley. One way to encourage pets to get more fluids is to add water to their dry

Call the Vet

Constipation that lasts longer than 48 hours can be serious because the stools get harder, drier, and bigger, until they don't have a chance of moving at all, says H. Ellen Whiteley, D.V.M., a veterinary consultant in Guadalupita, New Mexico, and consultant for *The Country Vet's Home Remedies for Cats.*

"Some pets start vomiting," she says. If that happens or if your pet becomes lethargic after being constipated for more than two days, see a veterinarian right away.

food. Better yet, moisten the food with low-salt chicken broth. Canned food is also a good source of fluids.

Dogs gladly drink water from a bowl, but some cats may have other preferences, Dr. Whiteley adds. "Make sure your cats have water available the way they like it, by leaving the faucet dripping, for example," she says. "That may encourage them to drink more."

Ask about enemas. Most pets won't need heroic measures to relieve constipation, but sometimes stools in the intestine get so dry and hard that they won't come out on their own. That's when your vet may recommend a natural enema, says Dr. Stefanatos. Enemas can be dangerous to give at home, so ask your vet for advice.

Groom away constipation. During grooming, cats swallow a lot of hair, which may form large clogs and cause constipation, says Dr. Stefanatos. You can usually prevent this by combing or brushing your cat every day—or by giving him a summer haircut. She recommends the "lion cut," in which you leave a mane and tuft of fur on the tail and clip the rest of the coat short.

Dehydration

The Signs

- Your pet's skin loses elasticity.
- His gums are sticky, and the saliva is stringy.
- His eyes are sunken.

Water makes up more than 90 percent of your pet's weight. Dogs and cats that lose as little as 10 percent of their internal water can get extremely ill from dehydration.

Healthy pets drink all the water they need to replace the fluids lost by panting, urinating, or having the occasional bouts of diarrhea and vomiting. But pets with illnesses such as kidney disease or diabetes may lose more fluid than they are able to take in. Severe vomiting or diarrhea can also cause dehydration. So can bacterial infections, which heat the body and speed the loss of essential fluids, says George Carley, D.V.M., a holistic veterinarian in private practice in Tulsa, Oklahoma.

Dehydration is always an emergency. If you suspect that your pet has lost a lot of fluids, test for dehydration by lifting and releasing the loose skin over the shoulders. If it doesn't snap back into place right away, your pet is probably dehydrated. Get him to a veterinarian immediately.

Veterinarians treat dehydration with large amounts of fluids, intravenously or under the skin. Once your pet's fluid levels are back to normal, however, holistic veterinarians look for ways to keep the body's fluids in balance naturally. Here is what they recommend.

The Solutions

Give him wet foods. The drawback to dry kibble is that it pulls water from the body to aid in digestion, says Anne Lampru, D.V.M., a holistic veterinarian in private practice in Tampa, Florida. This is more of a problem in cats because they get most of their water from food. Giving your pet moist food or adding water to his kibble will help ensure that he gets all the fluids he needs, she says.

Slow fluid loss with homeopathy. Diarrhea and vomiting are common causes of dehydration. A homeopathic remedy called Nux vomica quickly settles the stomach and intestines, helping ensure that water in the body stays there, says Kathleen Carson, D.V.M., a holistic veterinarian in private practice in Hermosa Beach, California. She recommends diluting 20 drops of Nux vomica 6C in an ounce of water and giving your pet half a dropperful three times a day until he is feeling better.

Many homeopathic remedies can be mixed in drinking water, but pets that are dehydrated probably won't drink enough to get the benefits. It is best to squirt the remedy directly in their mouths, using a needleless syringe or a medicine dropper, Dr. Carson says.

Restore their appetites. Dehydrated pets often refuse to eat, and this can make the problem worse, says James R. Richards, D.V.M., director of the Cornell Feline Health Center at Cornell University in Ithaca, New York. He recommends warming your pet's food before putting it in his bowl. Warming makes food smell stronger, and the smellier it is, the more likely your pet will eat it.

Encourage him to drink. Mild dehydration can often be reversed by encouraging your pet to drink plain water. One way to do this is to add a little low-salt chicken broth to his water or give him ice cubes. Many pets enjoy crunching ice, which will get more water into their systems, says Jory Olsen, D.V.M., a veterinary internal-medicine specialist in private practice in Marietta, Georgia. If your pet refuses to drink, your vet may recommend using a needleless syringe, loaded with plain water or a rehydration fluid such as Pedialyte, to put the liquid directly in his mouth.

Dental Problems

The Signs

- Your pet has smelly breath.
- The teeth are yellow or brown.
- He is chewing only on one side.
- He is drooling a lot or refusing to eat.

Almost all dogs and cats 3 years and older develop dental problems. What's to blame is plaque, a thin, bacteria-packed film that's a common cause of periodontal, or gum, disease. It can also lead to cavities, especially in cats, says Ihor Basko, D.V.M., a holistic veterinarian in private practice in Honolulu and Kilauea, Hawaii. More worrisome is that bacteria in the mouth sometimes slip into the bloodstream, damaging the heart or kidneys, he adds.

Veterinary dentists can repair some of the damage caused by dental disease, but the procedures are uncomfortable as well as expensive. But unlike many health threats, dental disease can often be stopped entirely with natural home care. It is not enough to just keep the teeth clean, Dr. Basko adds. You also have to strengthen the whole body so that your pet can fight dental disease from the inside out. Here's what veterinarians advise.

The Solutions

Give them foods with the perfect crunch. Dry kibble is supposed to cut down on dental problems by gently scrubbing the teeth. But most pets eat kibble in gulps, without a lot of chewing. It also tends to shatter when pets bite, so it doesn't really clean the teeth, says Anne Lampru, D.V.M., a holistic veterinarian in private practice in Tampa, Florida.

A better idea is to give your pet tartar-control foods and treats along with his regular food. They contain tough vegetable fibers, so when your pet takes a bite, the food particles literally wrap around the teeth, cleaning them with each bite, says Susan G. Wynn, D.V.M., a veterinarian in Atlanta and coeditor of *Complementary and Alternative Veterinary Medicine*. Tartar-control foods are available from vets. One good treat is TartarChek.

Give a healing enzyme. Pets with dental disease often have red, swollen, or bleeding gums. A naturally occurring enzyme called coenzyme Q_{10} helps gums heal more quickly, says Dr. Basko. He recommends giving cats and dogs weighing up to 20 pounds 10 milligrams of coenzyme Q_{10} a day. Dogs weighing 21 to 50 pounds can take up to 30 milligrams once a day, and dogs over 50 pounds can take 30 milligrams twice a day. You can stop the supplement when your pet's gums return to normal. Coenzyme Q_{10} is available in health food stores.

Increase immunity with vitamin C. The immune system is designed to fight bacteria throughout the body, including in the mouth. Vitamin C can help keep the immune system strong, says Dr. Basko. He recommends giving cats 100 to 250 milligrams of vitamin C a day. Dogs up to 50 pounds can take between 250 and 500 milligrams

Clean and White

The best way to keep your pet's breath fresh is to remove plaque from the teeth as soon as it appears. Here are products veterinarians recommend.

Pet toothpaste comes in tasty flavors like chicken, fish, liver, and malt. It won't upset your pet's stomach the way human toothpastes can. Be aware that antibacterial additives like chlorhexidine can be hard on the liver; discuss this with your vet. A safe alternative is baking soda with just enough hydrogen peroxide added to make a paste.

Finger brushes look like thimbles with bristles. Because they slip over the end of a finger, they are easy to use. A soft baby toothbrush also works fine. Or you can simply rub the outer surfaces of your pet's teeth with a piece of gauze. (The motion of the tongue keeps the inner surfaces clean.)

Dental floss chews are made of durable nylon strands that have been wrapped and tied in a knot. These toys remove plaque from between the teeth and at the gum line—and many dogs love them.

Rawhide chews often last for weeks, and the scraping action helps keep the teeth clean. Some rawhide chews are basted in spearmint for additional bad-breath control. Supervise your pet while he chews these so that he doesn't swallow large pieces.

Rubber-studded chews like Hercules and Rhino are made of extra-strong rubber and are covered with rubber teeth, which clean your pet's teeth and massage the gums while your pet chews.

a day, and those over 50 pounds can take 500 milligrams two or three times a day. Since vitamin C can cause diarrhea, you may have to cut back the dose until you find an amount your pet will tolerate.

Help them chew away plaque. A bone is nature's toothbrush, says Dr. Lampru, who recommends giving dogs and cats a bone to chew every day. It is important to use raw or lightly cooked (steamed for 15 to 30 seconds) bones because bones that are well-done splinter too easily, she adds.

For dogs, large knuckle bones are the best choice, and lightly steamed chicken necks are fine for cats, says Dr. Basko. A large dog or a determined cat may splinter even a tough bone, so make sure that the bone is too large to swallow and too tough to break down into fragments. Watch your pet chew. If he seems bent on destruction, give him a Kong or Nylabone instead.

Raw vegetables also rub away plaque, Dr. Basko adds. He recommends giving dogs and cats small bits of carrots, broccoli, or other vegetables and fruits several times a week. If your pet won't eat raw vegetables, lightly steam them.

Give them steak instead of hamburger. Many holistic veterinarians recommend giving pets raw meat as part of their daily diet. The problem with hamburger or chopped meat, however, is that it doesn't do a lot to keep the teeth clean. When meat is on the menu, says Dr. Basko, give your cat a large piece. You can also give your cat chicken gizzards to clean his teeth. Give dogs over 15 pounds a large, tough cut of beef that can't be swallowed whole. As pets chew off swallowable bits, they scour their teeth at the same time.

Some vets recommend lightly steaming the meat in order to kill harmful organisms such as salmonella, says

Allen M. Schoen, D.V.M., director of the Veterinary Institute for Therapeutic Alternatives in Sherman, Connecticut, and author of *Love, Miracles, and Animal Healing*.

Help with a supplement. Lactoferrin, available in capsule form, may be helpful for cats with gum disease. When the gums are inflamed, give between one-half and one 350-milligram capsule once a day, says Dr. Wynn. She recommends mixing the contents of the capsule in milk or syrup before giving it to your pet.

Diarrhea

The Signs

- Your pet's stools are soft and watery.
- She is having accidents in the house.

Anything that upsets the digestive tract, from eating garbage to having intestinal parasites, can cause diarrhea. In addition, some pets are allergic to ingredients in popular pet foods, which can also cause loose stools, explains Kathleen Carson, D.V.M., a holistic veterinarian in private practice in Hermosa Beach, California. And in some cases, pets can't digest properly because the foods don't contain the same enzymes that are found in natural whole foods.

Veterinarians occasionally use medications to stop diarrhea, although they usually recommend letting it run its course. The problem is that diarrhea may come back again and again. That is why holistic veterinarians try to get to the source of the problem. For many pets, this may be as simple as changing what goes in the food bowl. Along with a variety of natural remedies, changes in diet often stop diarrhea and prevent it from coming back.

The Solutions

Start with a fast. The quickest way to stop diarrhea is to put your pet on a food fast for 24 hours. When food isn't going into the intestines, nothing will come out, says H. Ellen Whiteley, D.V.M., a veterinary consultant in Guadalupita, New Mexico, and consultant for *The Country Vet's Home Remedies for Cats*. After a daylong fast, give your pet bland foods, such as skinless, boneless chicken breasts for cats and hamburger and rice for dogs. Keep the meals very small, and give them often, up to five or six times a day, she says. Fasting doesn't include taking away water, so keep the water bowl full. And check with your vet before putting young or diabetic pets on a fast.

Call the Vet

Diarrhea that comes on suddenly usually goes away just as quickly. But sometimes diarrhea is a sign of serious problems like distemper, parvovirus, or even poisoning, says H. Ellen Whiteley, D.V.M., a veterinary consultant in Guadalupita, New Mexico, and consultant for *The Country Vet's Home Remedies for Cats*.

When diarrhea is accompanied by blood in the stool or lasts more than 24 hours, call your vet. "Puppies and kittens can get dehydrated very quickly, and they may need fluid therapy and other supportive care," she adds.

Stop the discomfort with Nux vomica. This homeopathic remedy is good for the entire digestive tract and helps stop diarrhea, says Dr. Carson. She recommends using a 6X potency, mixing 20 drops in an ounce of spring water. Give your pet half a dropperful three times a day.

Stop the cramps. Dogs and cats with diarrhea often have painful cramps when the intestines expand and contract. A quick way to stop cramping is with aromatherapy, using an antispasmodic oil such as basil or peppermint, says Joanne Stefanatos, D.V.M., a holistic veterinarian in private practice in Las Vegas. She recommends diluting either of these essential oils half-and-half with vegetable oil and rubbing the mixture on the tips of your pet's ears until he is feeling better.

Put bacteria to work. The digestive tract always has a mixture of good and bad bacteria—and sometimes the bad wins, causing diarrhea. You can restore the body's natural

The Healing Instinct

"Eating dirt—a condition called pica—is common in dogs and cats," says H. Ellen Whiteley, a veterinary consultant in Guadalupita, New Mexico, and consultant for *The Country Vet's Home Remedies for Cats*. They don't do it because they love the taste. Researchers have found that certain soils can absorb harmful toxins in the intestine, buffer acidic foods, and replace essential minerals—all of which can be very helpful for pets with diarrhea.

If your pet just occasionally snacks on soil, she is probably just trying to keep her insides calm. A pet that does it all the time, however, probably has a problem and needs to see a vet.

balance by giving your pet additional beneficial bacteria. Try pet supplements containing *Lactobacillus acidophilus*, available in pet stores. Follow the label instructions. Or use live-culture yogurt, which contains the same organisms, Dr. Whiteley explains. Cats can have 1 to 2 teaspoons of yogurt a day, spread over several feedings. Dogs can take 1 to 2 tablespoons, depending on their size, she says.

Feed your pet a natural diet. "Changing to a good-quality food relieves some of the stress on the gut," says Dr. Carson. It also allows you to alter the ingredients according to your pet's needs. Your best strategy is to prepare your pet's meals at home, using whole ingredients like chicken, beef, rice, and fresh vegetables. Or buy an all-natural commercial food, like PetGuard Premium, she suggests.

Give your pet Kaopectate. Available in drugstores and supermarkets, Kaopectate contains a mineral found in clay that absorbs diarrhea-causing bacteria and toxins in the digestive tract. For pets under 15 pounds, Dr. Stefanatos recommends giving ½ teaspoon of Kaopectate every hour for 4 hours. Pets 15 to 50 pounds can take a teaspoon every hour, and dogs over 50 pounds can take a tablespoon every hour.

Firm the stools with fiber. Dietary fiber absorbs a lot of water in the digestive tract, which can help stop diarrhea, Dr. Stefanatos says. She recommends giving about ½ teaspoon of fiber-rich foods, such as flaxseeds or canned pumpkin, with every meal to cats and dogs weighing less than 15 pounds. Dogs 15 to 50 pounds can take a teaspoon of high-fiber foods, and larger dogs can take a tablespoon.

Ear Infections

The Signs
- Your pet shakes her head or holds it to one side.
- She scratches or rubs her ears, or she rubs her head against the furniture or carpet.
- There is a yellow, brown, or black discharge in one or both ears.
- The ears smell bad or are tender or red.

Dogs and cats have L-shaped ear canals, which helps prevent damage to their sensitive eardrums. The problem is this design allows the ears to trap moisture, debris, earwax, and parasites—any one of which can lead to ear infections. Cats often get infections because of ear mites, and up to 80 percent of ear problems in dogs are linked to allergies, adds Allen M. Schoen, D.V.M., director of the Veterinary Institute for Therapeutic Alternatives in Sherman, Connecticut, and author of *Love, Miracles, and Animal Healing.*

The traditional treatment is antibiotics, antifungal drugs, or other medications. But medications upset the normal chemistry inside the ear, possibly turning a simple infection into a complicated, long-term problem, says Ihor Basko, D.V.M., a holistic veterinarian in private practice in Honolulu and Kilauea, Hawaii. It makes more sense, he says, to deal with underlying allergies and strengthen the immune system so it can battle bacteria and other germs before they cause infection. In addition, there are many natural treatments for cleaning the ears and stopping infections without using drugs.

The Solutions

Clean the ears with vinegar. If your pet's ears are filled with brownish pink wax, there is a good chance that allergies have triggered a yeast infection. You can clear up yeast infections by cleaning the ears thoroughly. Veterinarians often recommend white vinegar, also called acetic acid, because it removes dirt and debris and helps restore a healthful chemical balance in the ears, says Anne Lampru, D.V.M., a holistic veterinarian in private practice in Tampa, Florida.

Diluted vinegar works well, but veterinarians often recommend a prescription product called Alocetic. It contains acetic acid along with aloe vera to soothe inflammation. When using either vinegar or Alocetic, pour a small amount into the ear canal, massage the area, then gently wipe the inside of the ear with a cotton ball. Do this once a day until the ear is better.

Stop infections with pau d'arco. Also called Inca Gold, the herb pau d'arco is a natural antibiotic that quickly kills fungi and bacteria, says Joanne Stefanatos, D.V.M., a holistic veterinarian in private practice in Las Vegas. Mix

Call the Vet

Ear infections usually affect only the outer part of the ear and aren't too serious. You should still see your veterinarian, however, to find out what is causing the problem, particularly if your pet is doing a lot of scratching. Vigorous scratching can break blood vessels in the earflap, causing the entire ear to swell like a balloon. It must be drained by a veterinarian to prevent permanent damage.

Watch out for head tilting, clumsiness, walking in circles, or drooping eyes. These are signs of an inner-ear infection, which must be treated by a vet. Your pet will probably need antibiotics to knock out the infection. In addition, your vet may need to drain pus and other fluids from inside the ear.

equal parts pau d'arco (*Tabebuia impetiginosa*) tincture and mineral oil, and put several drops in your pet's ears at the first sign of infection, she says. You can give the drops two or three times a day for several days.

Reduce inflammation with vitamin C. The adrenal glands produce a natural steroid that can help reduce inflammation when ears get infected. Giving pets vitamin C can help the adrenal glands work more efficiently. Cats and dogs weighing under 15 pounds can take between 100 and 250 milligrams of vitamin C a day. Pets 15 to 50 pounds can take 250 to 500 milligrams a day, and larger dogs can take 500 milligrams two or three times a day, says Dr. Basko. Vitamin C can cause diarrhea, so you may have to cut back the dose until you find an amount that your pet will tolerate.

Eliminate toxins with a healthful diet. Giving your pet a healthful, homemade diet or high-quality commercial food that doesn't contain additives or preservatives can vastly reduce the amount of wax that the ears produce while also helping the immune system work well, explains Dr. Basko.

Air out the ears. Increasing air circulation inside the ears can control the growth of bacteria, yeast, and fungi, says Dr. Lampru. Periodically trim around the opening of the ear canal with blunt-nosed scissors or electric clippers so the hair is about ½-inch long. Plucking excess hair inside the ears also allows air to circulate. Plucking can be painful, however, so vets recommend having it done by a groomer.

Strengthen the digestive tract. Supplements such as bromelain and quercetin can help prevent an allergic response in the gastrointestinal tract, making food allergies less of a problem, says Dr. Schoen. While your pet has the infection, give a 250-milligram quercetin/bromelain combination capsule (like Doctor's Best) 15 to 30 minutes before each meal. You can give pets weighing less than 15 pounds one-quarter capsule. Pets weighing 15 to 50 pounds can take one-half to one whole capsule. And larger dogs can take one to two capsules, he says.

Stop ear mites with oil. When an infection is caused by ear mites, putting a few drops of almond or olive oil in each ear will smother the mites and may allow the infection to heal, explains Dr. Lampru. You usually need to continue the oil treatments for 3 to 4 weeks, putting 3 to 7 drops of oil into the ear canals each day. Cleaning wax and other debris from the ears before using oil helps the treatment work more efficiently.

Try an over-the-counter remedy. Products containing pyrethrins, like Natural Animal and Pet Gold herbal powders, are helpful for ear mites. Made from chrysanthemums, pyrethrins are natural insecticides that are very safe to use, says Dr. Lampru. Just follow the directions on the label.

Ear Mites

The Signs
- Your pet scratches her ears all the time.
- There is dark, dry debris in the ears.
- Her ears are inflamed or swollen.

The insides of your pet's ears are warm, moist, and well-protected—and provide a perfect environment for mites. These annoying creatures are so small that you can barely see them, but your pets can certainly feel them. Ear mites—and the nonstop itching they cause—can result in sores, infections, or even hearing loss, says Carolyn Blakey, D.V.M., a holistic veterinarian in private practice in Richmond, Indiana. Dogs occasionally get ear mites, but it is generally more of a problem in cats, she adds.

You can eliminate ear mites with medications, but the mites may come back, usually when the body's natural defenses are weaker than they should be. In most cases, how-

ever, there are gentle, more natural ways to get rid of them
and to keep them from coming back.

The Solutions

Start with a tea rinse. Green tea is a natural antiseptic
that helps remove "mite mess" from the ear canal, says
Michele Yasson, D.V.M., a holistic veterinarian in private
practice in New York City and Rosendale, New York.
Steep a tablespoon of green tea leaves in a cup of hot
water for 3 to 4 minutes, strain it, then let it cool to room
temperature. Using a small dropper, flush your pet's ear
canal with the tea. Massage the outside of the ear to circulate the tea, then stand back: When your pet shakes her
head, the tea—along with the grit in the ear—will come
flying out. Then dry the outer part of the ear canal with a
tissue or cotton ball, says Dr. Yasson. Do this once a day
for a month.

Foil them with oil. A traditional all-natural remedy for
mites is to put 3 to 5 drops of oil in the ear canal. The oil

Easy Ear Drops

To give your cat ear drops without getting scratched,
wrap her entire body, including the feet, securely in a
small bath towel. Leave her head unwrapped and make
sure that the towel is loose enough for her to breathe.
Circle her head with your hand, putting your fingers
under her chin and your thumb over the top of her head
to hold her steady. With the other hand, hold the ear
dropper so that the opening is just above the ear canal.
Put in the drops and massage the base of her ear to
circulate the liquid.

smothers the mites and also helps soothe the ears, says Dr. Yasson. Generally, it doesn't matter what kind of oil you use, although some holistic vets recommend almond or olive oil. (Don't use tea tree oil, which can be dangerous for cats.) For a double benefit, soak a few crushed garlic cloves in the oil overnight. Garlic helps kill bacteria that can lead to ear infections in pets with ear mites, says Dr. Yasson. Give the oil treatments once a day for at least a month, she adds.

For the oil to be effective, clean your pet's ears first. Otherwise, the accumulated discharge may protect the mites from the oil.

Help the body help itself. Once you have gotten rid of ear mites, make sure they don't come back. Some holistic veterinarians recommend echinacea (*Echinacea purpurea* or *Echinacea angustifolia*), an herb that strengthens the immune system and makes it harder for parasites to thrive.

Call the Vet

Ear mites rarely cause serious problems—unless your pet scratches her ears so vigorously that she damages the skin or gets an infection.

It is fine to try home remedies for about a month, says Michele Yasson, D.V.M., a holistic veterinarian in private practice in New York City and Rosendale, New York. If your pet is still scratching, see your vet for more powerful treatments to kill the mites and stop the itching.

Don't wait a month, however, if your pet also has swelling inside the ear or a pus-filled or discolored discharge, she adds. These are signs of infection, so see the vet right away.

Give echinacea for about 2 weeks after treating your pet for mites.

Dogs and cats usually take echinacea liquid without putting up a fuss, but some pets dislike the taste. An alternative is echinacea capsules. Either way, give dogs over 50 pounds the full human dose, says Dr. Yasson. Pets 20 to 50 pounds can take one-half the human dose, and pets under 20 pounds should take one-quarter the human dose.

Feed them well. High-quality foods—or nutritious, homemade foods—keep the immune system strong and help prevent mites from getting established, says Dr. Yasson.

Treat all your pets. One reason mites are so hard to get rid of is that they are readily passed from pet to pet, says Dr. Yasson. Even if you successfully treat one pet, she may get reinfected the next time that she rubs heads with one of her friends. The only way to get rid of mites for good is to treat all your pets—not just the one that's doing the scratching.

Eye Irritation

The Signs

- Your pet's eyes are red, itchy or inflamed.
- There is a yellow or green discharge in the corner of the eye.
- Her eyes continually water.
- The skin around the eyes is swollen.
- She squints or won't open one eye.

The eyes are a lot tougher than they look. Dogs and cats are always coming into contact with something—from the sharp tip of a foxtail to irritating pollen in the air—that causes one or both eyes to swell, water, or redden, a condition called conjunctivitis.

Most eye irritations aren't serious and go away on their own within a few days. But it is impossible to tell at home which irritations are minor and which are scary. You really need to call your vet when you notice any problems with the eyes, says Steve Marsden, N.D., D.V.M., a naturopathic physician and holistic veterinarian in private practice in Beaverton, Oregon.

Fortunately, some cases of eye irritation are easy to treat at home. Veterinarians who specialize in holistic medicine have developed a number of simple, drug-free strategies that stop pain and inflammation quickly. Here are their tips.

The Solutions

Brighten the eyes with eyebright. This herb (*Euphrasia officinalis*) is an antioxidant and anti-inflammatory that nourishes and eases irritated eyes, says Betsy Walker Harrison, D.V.M., a holistic veterinarian in private practice in Wimberley, Texas. She recommends mixing 5 drops of eyebright extract in a cup of saline solution and putting a few drops in each of your pet's eyes. (Hold your pet's head

Help for Dry Eyes

Some pets, especially dogs, develop dry eye, a condition in which there aren't enough tears to keep the eyes lubricated. Veterinarians have always believed that there isn't a cure. The main treatment was to use artificial tears, a sterile fluid that resembles the body's natural tears, or to give a drug called cyclosporine, which increases tear production and can slow the destruction of the tear gland. But some holistic veterinarians believe that dry eye is associated with liver problems, says Steve Marsden, N.D., D.V.M., a naturopathic physician and holistic veterinarian in private practice in Beaverton, Oregon. When the liver problems are taken care of, the eyes often take care of themselves, he explains.

securely, and place the dropper directly over her eye but not touching it. Hold the eye open with one hand while squeezing in the drops with the other.) Or you can soak a gauze pad in the solution and use it to gently swab her eyes once or twice a day.

Eyebright also works as a compress. Steep an eyebright tea bag in a cup of warm water for 5 minutes. Let it cool, then use the tea to moisten a soft, clean cloth. Gently hold the damp cloth across your pet's eyes. You can apply the compress twice a day for 3 to 5 minutes at a time.

Stop the sting. A quick way to reduce eye pain and swelling is to combine equal parts eyebright and goldenseal eyedrops, both of which can be purchased, and put 1 or 2 drops of the solution in your pet's eyes three times a day, says Dr. Marsden.

Coat the eyes. Another way to ease irritation quickly is to put one drop of almond or cod-liver oil in your pet's eyes one to four times a day, says Dr. Harrison.

Help injuries heal. Dogs and cats sometimes get minor eye injuries that can cause painful irritation, says Dr. Harrison. These homeopathic remedies can be very effective.

- Arnica is recommended when tissues surrounding the eye are inflamed or swollen.
- Symphytum is good when the eyeball has taken a direct hit.
- Belladonna stops inflammation and is often recommended for pinkeye.
- Pulsatilla is used when pets have pinkeye as well as thick yellow or greenish discharge.
- Euphrasia helps pets that are tearing heavily.

Whichever remedy you use, veterinarians usually suggest giving two 30C pellets. Give one dose and wait a half-hour, advises Dr. Harrison. If the eye still isn't better, give a second dose.

Call the Vet

Here are four signs that *always* mean you should call
the vet, says Steve Marsden, N.D., D.V.M., a naturopathic physician and holistic veterinarian in private
practice in Beaverton, Oregon. Don't bother with home
care, says Dr. Marsden. "Go straight to your vet."

- The eye is clearly painful, and your pet is shaking
  her head or pawing her eye to get relief.
- The blood vessels in the whites of the eyes (the
  sclera) are unusually swollen.
- The main part of the eye, the cornea, has unusual
  lines or circles, or it appears to be layered.
- The entire eye suddenly becomes cloudy.

Give them chrysanthemum. Any species of chrysanthemum sold as the Chinese remedy juhua is good for relieving eye irritation, Dr. Marsden says. He recommends
giving cats and dogs under 15 pounds ¼ teaspoon of the
powdered herb twice a day. Pets 15 to 50 pounds can take
½ teaspoon, and larger dogs can have up to 1 tablespoon.

Feline Immunodeficiency Virus

The Signs
- Your cat has a fever that comes and goes.
- The lymph nodes—under the jaw and elsewhere— are swollen.
- He has sores in his mouth.
- He refuses to eat and is losing weight.
- He keeps getting infections.

It has been called feline AIDS because the virus that causes it is closely related to the human virus. Cats that get feline immunodeficiency virus, or FIV, often have no symptoms at all. It often takes up to 6 years before cats with FIV get sick, if they get sick at all.

The virus weakens the entire immune system, making cats vulnerable to secondary illnesses, in which otherwise minor conditions like diarrhea or runny eyes begin causing problems.

There isn't a cure for FIV, but there is a lot you can do

to ensure that your cat, even if infected, has a long, healthy life. "The best treatment is to keep their immune systems as healthy and strong as possible," says Pat Zook, D.V.M., a holistic veterinarian in private practice in Stone Mountain, Georgia.

The Solutions

Give your cat wheat sprouts. They contain compounds that act as immunity-building antioxidants, says Dr. Zook. She recommends Feline Support, which contains wheat sprout derivatives along with a variety of antioxidants. You can give your cat one wheat sprout supplement a day. Some cats crunch them right down, but others won't touch them unless you crush them first and mix them in their food.

Give an herbal boost. The herb astragalus (*Astragalus membranaceus*), available as a tincture, gives the immune system a long-term boost, says Dr. Zook. She recommends giving cats 4 drops of the tincture twice a day. Herbal tinctures that contain alcohol aren't good for long-term use, she adds. Look for glycerin-based tinctures in health food stores.

Cool fevers. Fever helps the body fight infections, but it can be dangerous for cats with FIV because they are already weakened. One way to lower fever is to dab a little rubbing alcohol on the pads of the feet. Alcohol stings, so don't use it if your cat has cuts or sores on his feet, says Alice Wolf, D.V.M., professor of medicine at Texas A&M University College of Veterinary Medicine in College Station.

Feed him well. Good nutrition is vital for cats with FIV. Holistic veterinarians recommend a homemade diet of one-half meat, one-quarter raw vegetables, and one-quarter cooked carbohydrates, like brown rice. Or give your cat a high-quality, all-natural pet food like Innova or

Solid Gold, says Carolyn Blakey, D.V.M., a holistic veterinarian in private practice in Richmond, Indiana.

Give natural enzymes. To help your cat get the most nutrients from his food, give him a raw egg yolk once a week and a teaspoon of nonflavored live-culture yogurt five days a week. These foods may contain natural enzymes, which will help the digestive system work more efficiently, says Roger L. DeHaan, D.V.M., a holistic veterinarian in private practice in Frazee, Minnesota. You can also give your cat a commercial digestive enzyme for pets, such as Prozyme or FloraZyme; follow the directions on the label.

Provide extra vitamins. Give cats with FIV antioxidants—vitamins C, E, and A—to help boost the immune system, says Dr. Blakey. She recommends a combination supplement, available from veterinarians, called Cell-Advance 440. Give your cat one capsule a day, she advises.

Fever

The Signs
- Your pet is panting even when he is resting.
- The ears are hot and may be red inside.
- His appetite is off.
- His energy level is low.

While prolonged high temperatures can be a problem, most fevers aren't dangerous. In fact, they may help pets recover because they make it more difficult for germs to thrive inside the body.

The conventional approach is to give medications that fight infection and lower fever. But vets who practice natural healing feel it is equally important to bolster the immune system at the same time. Of course, even a slight fever can make pets feel hot and miserable. Here are a few ways to lower the heat and help your pet fight off the underlying problem.

The Solutions

Cook some comfort food. Pets with fevers often lose their appetites, so they run short on nutrients. They also tend to quit drinking fluids, which raises the risk of dehydration. Putting a little sodium-free chicken or beef broth in their bowls encourages them to lap up critical fluids along with vitamins and minerals, says Maria H. Glinski, D.V.M., a holistic veterinarian in private practice in Glendale, Wisconsin.

For cats, a bowl of tuna juice is hard to resist. Squeeze the liquid from a can of tuna into a bowl and dilute it half-

Call the Vet

Fever may be a sign of serious problems, says Maria H. Glinski, D.V.M., a holistic veterinarian in private practice in Glendale, Wisconsin. "We worry most when the fever is in a very young or very old animal because they are more fragile and dehydrate more easily."

The normal temperature for dogs is between 100° and 102.5°F. For cats, it is between 101° and 102.5°. Check it with a rectal thermometer. Lubricate the end of a pet thermometer with petroleum jelly and gently twirl it into the rectum. Insert it no more than 1 inch in cats and small dogs, 2 inches in medium and large dogs. Hold your pet still for about 2 minutes, then remove the thermometer and check the reading. A fever of 103.5° or higher is potentially dangerous, and you should call your vet right away.

If your pet has other symptoms—he is vomiting, for example, or hasn't eaten for 24 hours or more—don't wait to see whether the temperature is rising or not. Call your vet right away.

and-half with water, says Susan G. Wynn, D.V.M., a veterinarian in Atlanta and coeditor of *Complementary and Alternative Veterinary Medicine.*

Put herbs to work. Echinacea (*Echinacea angustifolia* or *Echincacea purpurea*) helps the body fight infection, says herbalist Gregory L. Tilford, co-owner of Animals' Apawthecary in Conner, Montana, and author of *Edible and Medicinal Plants of the West.* He recommends giving pets with a fever 12 to 20 drops of a low- or non-alcohol echinacea tincture for every 20 pounds of weight. Give the drops two or three times a day, he says.

Another herb that can boost immunity is astragalus (*Astragalus membranaceus*). Use it in the same amounts as echinacea, Tilford says.

Try some Hepar sulphuris calcareum. Also known as Hepar sulph, this homeopathic remedy helps reduce fevers caused by a variety of infections, says Dr. Glinski. She recommends a 6C or 30C pellet. Give one pellet to pets under 50 pounds and two pellets to larger dogs. Repeat the treatment once an hour for 4 hours, she advises.

Provide some puncture protection. It is not uncommon for pets to develop fevers from infected puncture wounds. The homeopathic remedy for this type of infection is Ledum—one dose of either 6C or 30C pellets. When pets are given the remedy immediately after their injuries, germs are much less likely to cause infections, abscesses, or fever, says Linda East, D.V.M., a holistic veterinarian in private practice in Denver. You can give two pellets of Ledum to dogs over 50 pounds and one pellet to smaller pets.

Relieve the aches and pains. Fever can make pets feel sore all over. To ease the aches, Dr. Glinski recommends the homeopathic remedy Arnica. Give one 30C pellet to pets under 15 pounds and two pellets to larger pets. Repeat the treatment once an hour for up to 4 hours. It is not a good idea to mix homeopathic remedies, so be sure to use Arnica only after stopping Hepar sulph or Ledum.

Make him stronger with vitamin C. This powerhouse nutrient can help stimulate your pet's immune system so that it is better able to fight off viral and bacterial infections, says Dr. Glinski. She recommends mixing a little buffered, powdered vitamin C in a dollop of yogurt or cottage cheese. Most pets gulp it right down.

Dogs over 50 pounds can be given 1,000 milligrams twice a day, while smaller pets should take only 500 milligrams once a day. Just be sure not to give straight vitamin C, she warns. It contains ascorbic acid, which may upset your pet's stomach. In addition, large amounts of vitamin C may cause diarrhea, so it is a good idea to give smaller doses at first to give the body time to adjust.

Give them plenty of water. Feverish pets can become dehydrated very quickly. Keep their water bowls full, preferably with spring or filtered water. If your pet refuses to drink, fill an eyedropper or turkey baster with water and squirt a little into the side of his mouth. (Don't squirt the water toward the back of his mouth because it might get into the lungs.) For an added boost, offer your pet a bowl of electrolyte solution, such as Pedialyte, which restores essential minerals called electrolytes, Dr. Glinski says.

Brew some herbal pain relief. Willow bark tea (*Salix alba*), which, like aspirin, contains salicylates, can reduce fever and help ease aches and pains, Tilford says. (Aspirin and other substances containing salicylates may be harmful for cats and should never be used without a veterinarian's supervision.) Stir a teaspoon of shredded willow bark in 8 ounces of hot water and simmer for about 3 minutes. Let it cool to room temperature and give a tablespoon or 2 for every 20 pounds of pooch twice a day, he suggests.

Finicky Eating

The Signs

- Your pet refuses to eat or leaves large portions of his food untouched.
- He begs whenever you are eating.

Dogs and cats establish their tastes for food in the first months of life. Up to 6 months old, they eat almost anything. But after this, they tend to dislike novel tastes, and some adults will flatly refuse to eat unusual food. Old cats in particular may prefer to go hungry rather than try something new.

In most families, people and pets quickly arrive at mutually agreeable menus. Problems occur when pets, for no apparent reason, stop eating their dinners and start begging for something different. Once they get accustomed to receiving special treats, it's hard to get them eating normally again. And in the meantime, you'll have to put up with meows, moans, and perpetual mooching. It's not difficult to convince your pets to be less fussy, but it may take some time. Here's what experts advise.

The Solutions

Hang tough. What goes in their mouths is entirely up to you. If you hold tough, nix the fancy snacks, and give them only pet food for a few days, there's a good chance their fussy habits will disappear, says David McMillan, a trainer and owner of Worldwide Movie Animals in Canyon Country, California.

Make mealtime more social. Pets tend to be less finicky about their food when they're allowed to eat in the kitchen or dining room along with the rest of the family, says Diana Philips, a trainer and owner of Spirit of the Moon Animal Talent in Gibsonton, Florida.

Count to 15. Many pets, especially cats, are accustomed to free-choice feeding, in which food is available all the time. But sometimes food loses its appeal when pets have been looking at it all day, Smith says. A better approach is to put the food down for 15 minutes. If your pet hasn't eaten, pick up the food and put it away. If food is "scarce," your pet will probably value it more, she says.

Acknowledge her "tuna jones." Cats that crave a single food—usually tuna—may refuse to eat anything else. While a pure tuna diet isn't very good for cats, expecting them to go "cold tuna" is unrealistic because some will literally starve before eating something else, says Grant Nisson, D.V.M., a veterinarian at Muddy Creek Animal Hospital in West River, Maryland. Ease your cat into a new eating style by adding a little tuna to the food you want her to eat. Each day, add a little less tuna. Within a month or two, most cats will be eating normally again, he says.

Feed them late. The appetite is partly controlled by the body's natural rhythms, and some dogs and cats simply aren't ready to eat until 9 or 10 P.M. Late-night feedings are especially helpful in summer, when high temperatures can make dogs and cats reluctant to eat, says Ben Kersen, a trainer in Victoria, British Columbia.

Stimulate the appetite with exercise. Pets that are excited by life tend to eat more heartily than those that are lackadaisical, Kersen says. Exercise also burns calories, of course, which results in a heartier appetite. Veterinarians agree that healthy dogs and cats can easily use 20 minutes of vigorous play a day—all at once or, for older, less vigorous pets, in 5-minute increments.

Play hide-and-seek. For creatures that evolved as hunters, few things are more boring than a bowl of lifeless kibble. To stimulate your pet's senses along with her appetite, put the thrill back into eating by hiding small servings of food around the house and letting her sniff them out, says Joanne Howl, D.V.M., a veterinarian in West River, Maryland, and former president of the Maryland Veterinary Medical Association.

Warm their food. Food that's heated in the microwave or doused with a little warm water releases more aromas than cold foods and is more appealing, Smith says. Don't make it too hot, however, because some pets will gulp food even when it's scalding hot.

Nip it in the nest. Dogs and cats establish many of their habits when they're young. To keep them from getting picky later on, expose them to a wide variety of foods. Switch brands now and then. Give them chicken flavor instead of beef flavor. You may even want to give them small tastes of fruit, vegetables, and cheese, Dr. Nisson says. The idea is to help them understand that new foods are also good foods.

Keep in mind, too, that fruits and vegetables are high in fiber and low in calories. If your puppy develops a fondness for crunchy carrots, apple slices, grapes, and sugar snap peas as treats, you could avoid a weight problem later on.

Flatulence

The Signs
- Your pet is passing gas every day.
- The odor is ruining your relationship.

Social implications aside, flatulence isn't a serious problem. "It is your pet's way of telling you that there is something indigestible in his diet," says Susan G. Wynn, D.V.M., a veterinarian in Atlanta and coeditor of *Complementary and Alternative Veterinary Medicine.*

Even though occasional flatulence is normal, holistic veterinarians believe too much gas is a sign that your pet's diet and overall health aren't as good as they could be. Here are a few ways to clear the air and keep your pet more comfortable.

The Solutions
Feed him the wild way. Your pet's digestive tract is pretty much the same as his wild ancestors'. Some holistic vets believe that giving dogs and cats a "wild" diet will im-

prove their digestion while curtailing the fumes. Russell Swift, D.V.M., a holistic veterinarian in private practice in Dade, Broward, and Palm Beach Counties in Florida, recommends a diet that includes raw meat and vegetables, bonemeal, digestive enzymes, and beneficial bacteria such as acidophilus. Every pet has different nutritional needs, so ask your vet to help plan a healthful, low-gas diet.

Switch to a different food. Your pet will probably be less gassy if you give him a food that contains a higher percentage of meat-based protein, says Dr. Wynn. Look for foods in which proteins from meat sources constitute at least two of the first three ingredients listed on the label, she advises.

Put yogurt to work. Changing your pet's diet will often change the balance of bacteria in the intestine, causing a sudden increase in flatulence. To keep him smelling sweet, Dr. Wynn advises adding a little plain, live-culture yogurt to his food. This will reduce gas by replacing some of the good bacteria in the digestive tract. Give him yogurt for several days after changing his diet, she adds. Give 1 to 2 teaspoons of yogurt a day to pets under 15 pounds; dogs over 80 pounds can have up to 3 tablespoons a day. Middle-sized dogs can have proportionately less.

Use a yogurt substitute. While yogurt is good for most pets, some dogs and cats are sensitive to lactose, a sugar found in milk, yogurt, and other dairy foods. If your pet gets diarrhea after eating yogurt, use acidophilus supplements instead, says Jeffrey Feinman, V.M.D., a holistic veterinarian in private practice in Fairfield County in Connecticut. You can give pets over 15 pounds the human dose listed on the label; smaller pets can take half of the human dose, he says. Acidophilus supplements are available in supermarkets and health food stores.

Add a little water. Dry pet foods contain enormous amounts of air, which can cause flatulence. Soaking dry

Call the Vet

When intestinal gas occurs all the time or is accompanied by other symptoms like diarrhea, weight loss, or blood or mucus in the stool, there may be a problem in the digestive tract.

Severe flatulence is often a sign of parasites, says Jeffrey Feinman, V.M.D., a holistic veterinarian in private practice in Fairfield County in Connecticut. It can also be caused by a serious condition called inflammatory bowel disease. When flatulence doesn't go away within a day or two, call your vet, he says. This is especially true for cats since they are less likely to be gassy in the first place.

food in water until it triples in size removes the air before it gets into the digestive tract, Dr. Feinman says.

The one drawback to soaking dry food is that it loses some of its ability to scrape the teeth clean. A compromise is to soak most of the food, but sprinkle a little dry food on top, Dr. Feinman suggests.

Curb it with charcoal. Activated charcoal, available in health food stores and drugstores, can absorb tremendous amounts of gas in the digestive tract, says Dr. Swift. He recommends giving cats and small dogs (under 15 pounds) one-quarter of the dose listed on the label. Pets 15 to 50 pounds can take one-half of the recommended dose, and dogs over 50 pounds can take the full amount.

Purge it with papaya. To relieve flatulence caused by dietary indiscretions, such as rooting through the garbage, Dr. Feinman recommends papaya enzyme once a day for several days. Available in health food stores, papaya enzyme helps break down gas-producing particles in the digestive tract. A dog that weighs 50 pounds can take the dose for adults, he says. You can give more or less of the enzyme to larger or smaller dogs, depending on their weight.

Dr. Swift often recommends "broad-spectrum" digestive enzymes such as Prozyme, available from holistic veterinarians and pet supply stores. These enzymes help break down proteins, carbohydrates, fats, and fiber. Dr. Swift recommends sprinkling the enzyme on your pet's food; follow the instructions on the package.

Fleas

The Signs
- Your pet is scratching a lot or losing patches of fur.
- There is pepperlike debris in his fur.
- His skin is red or sore, or there is a scabby rash.
- He has been getting tapeworms.

Flea bites are painless and by themselves aren't always itchy. But many dogs and cats are allergic to flea saliva. A bite can trigger a scratching frenzy that can last as long as a week. Some pets get so itchy and scratch so hard that they damage the skin, causing a painful infection.

Most veterinarians have begun recommending medications to fight fleas. These products are very effective, but you may be able to control the problem without drugs or spray-on pesticides. "The holistic approach takes longer, but it uses less toxic approaches," says Nancy Scanlan, D.V.M., a holistic veterinarian in private practice in Sherman Oaks, California. Here are some natural recommendations.

The Solutions

Use a natural repellent. Keep fleas off your pet with a supplement called Body Guard Powder, available from some vets, says Joanne Stefanatos, D.V.M., a holistic veterinarian in private practice in Las Vegas. During flea season, pets weighing under 20 pounds can have 1 teaspoon twice a day, mixed in their food. Pets weighing 20 to 50 pounds can take 1½ teaspoons twice daily, and larger pets can take up to a tablespoon twice a day.

Repel them with bad taste. A combination of brewer's yeast and garlic changes the flavor of your pet's blood, making it unappealing to fleas, says Dr. Scanlan. She recommends sprinkling about a tablespoon of brewer's yeast on your pet's food each day. Dogs over 50 pounds can have as much as 2 teaspoons of garlic a day, and smaller dogs can have ¼ to ½ teaspoon a day. Garlic can be a problem for cats, so don't give them too much. A safe limit is ⅛ teaspoon or less a day for up to 2 weeks at a time. Some dogs are allergic to yeast, however, so it is a good idea to check with your vet before using it at home.

To Catch a Flea

Fill a cake pan with soapy water and put it under a night-light near where your pet sleeps. Fleas are attracted to light and will make a leap for it—and land in the water and drown.

Drive them off with bad smells. Fleas don't like the smell of citrus, and you can often keep them away by washing floors and baseboards with Lemon Fresh or cleaners that contain citronella, says Dr. Stefanatos.

Other aromatic herbs that repel fleas include pennyroyal (*Mentha pulegium* or *Hedeoma pulegioides*), peppermint (*Mentha piperita*), and spearmint (*Mentha spicata*), says Pat Zook, D.V.M., a holistic veterinarian in private practice in Stone Mountain, Georgia. Make an herbal tea by putting ¼ cup of the dried herb in a quart of hot water and letting it steep in a covered pot for 15 minutes. Strain the tea, let it cool, and mop it on your floors and baseboards.

Aromatic cedar is another natural flea repellent, says Carin A. Smith, D.V.M., a veterinary consultant in the state of Washington and author of *Get Rid of Fleas and Ticks for Good!*

Comb them out. "Use a flea comb to remove fleas from your pet every day," says Dr. Smith. "Comb your pet over a hard floor so that you can see and catch the fleas. Keep a bowl of soapy water nearby, and drop in the fleas to drown them."

Fill the tub. Give your pet a good dunking in a tub or sink all the way up to his neck, says Dr. Smith. The fleas will quickly head for dry ground above the neck, and you can pick them off as soon as they appear.

To make the bath even more effective, lather up your pet's neck with a flea shampoo containing pyrethrins, a natural insecticide made from chrysanthemums. Leave the lather on for about 10 minutes. When the fleas run uphill, they get trapped in the suds and die, Dr. Smith explains. Then rinse your pet thoroughly to send the remaining fleas down the drain.

Call the Vet

"Each flea drinks 15 times its body weight in blood every day," says Carin A. Smith, D.V.M., a veterinary consultant in the state of Washington and author of *Get Rid of Fleas and Ticks for Good!* When your pet has a lot of fleas—100 or more at a time isn't unusual—he can lose up to a milliliter of blood a day. This isn't a problem for grown, healthy pets, but it can cause anemia in puppies and kittens as well as in older pets that have other health problems.

You can recognize anemia by looking in your pet's mouth. The gums and tongue should be a healthy, bubble-gum pink. If they are pale or white, he could be losing large amounts of blood. Call your vet right away.

Hit them when they are down. A bath kills fleas, but it won't keep new ones off. So dust or spray your pet with a flea product containing pyrethrins, following the instructions on the label, Dr. Smith advises.

Dust with diatomaceous earth. It's a fine powder consisting of the skeletons of microscopic algae that contain trace minerals. It can help keep your pet's skin healthy so it naturally repels fleas, says Dr. Scanlan. Liberally sprinkle it on your pet once a day during flea season and rub it into the skin, she says.

You can buy diatomaceous earth in pet supply stores. Be sure to buy the kind called amorphous, Dr. Scanlan adds. Another type, called glassified, is used as a filter in swimming pools and can be dangerous for pets.

Stop the itch with homeopathy. To stop itching caused by fleas, give one to three pellets of the homeopathic remedy Ctenocephalidae nosode 12X three times day for 1 week, says Dr. Stefanatos.

Treat it with oatmeal. Washing pets with an oatmeal shampoo is one of the best ways to relieve itching, says Steven A. Melman, D.V.M., a veterinarian with practices in Potomac, Maryland, and Palm Springs, California, and author of *Skin Diseases of Dogs and Cats*. Be sure to use cool water because warm water makes itching worse, he adds. You can use the oatmeal shampoo once a day for 3 to 4 days.

Suck up the problem. For every adult flea on your pet, there may be 100 more eggs, larvae, and cocoons in the house. "Get rid of them by vacuuming your house at least once a week," says Dr. Smith. Be sure to vacuum the furniture, cracks in the baseboards, and other dark places where flea larvae wait to mature. Throw out the vacuum cleaner bag each week, she adds. Otherwise, the eggs inside the bag will hatch and start the problem all over again.

Wash his bedding. "Wash fabrics that your pet lies on at least once a week because normal washing in hot water and soap will remove flea eggs and larvae," says Dr. Smith. If your pet likes lounging on the furniture, cover it with towels, which you can change every day.

Salt the carpet. An all-natural substance called borax salts causes adult fleas to dry out and die. It also kills flea larvae when they eat or inhale the dust, says Dr. Scanlan. Look for sodium polyborate on the label; it's in products such as Rx for Fleas. Dr. Scanlan recommends working the powder deep into the carpet, then vacuuming up the residue. "Wear a mask when applying borax salts, and don't let pets onto the carpet until you have vacuumed up the excess," she adds. Borax salts are very effective, but the benefits are temporary: As soon as you shampoo the rug, you have to powder it again.

Put worms to work. To get rid of outdoor fleas waiting to attack your pet, Dr. Scanlan recommends nematodes, microscopic worms that you can get from garden supply stores. When mixed in water and sprayed on the yard, nematodes eat immature fleas as well as other insects, she explains.

Take away their hiding places. Fleas thrive in moist shaded areas—in tall grass, for example, or in weeds underneath trees. "One way to control fleas is to keep the grass mowed short," says Dr. Scanlan.

Hair Balls

The Signs
- Your pet is throwing up wads of hair.

Cats can spend hours a day busily engaged in grooming. What's good for their coats, however, isn't so good for their insides. With every lick, loose fur sticks to their rough tongues, so they swallow it. Some of the hair is eliminated in the stools, but some stays in the stomach, forming a gooey wad. When enough hair accumulates, cats chuck it up, leaving an unpleasant hairy mess—usually on your best carpet.

Hair balls occur mainly in cats, especially the long-haired breeds, but dogs, too, can get them.

Veterinarians sometimes advise giving pets an oily remedy, available in pet supply stores and from veterinarians, that lubricates the hair and helps it slide through the intestines. The problem is these types of products contain artificial flavors and preservatives. That is why holistic veterinarians prefer to use natural methods both for preventing hair balls and for eliminating those that have already formed.

The Solutions

Help them pass with petroleum jelly. Place about ¼ teaspoon of petroleum jelly on your pet's front paws. When he licks his paws, he will swallow the petroleum jelly, which will lubricate hairs in the stomach so that they move gently into the digestive tract. Apply the petroleum jelly once a day for about 4 days until your pet stops hacking, says Craig N. Carter, D.V.M., Ph.D., head of epidemiology at the Texas Veterinary Medical Diagnostic Laboratory at Texas A&M University in College Station.

Give them extra fiber. The dietary fiber found in food like canned pumpkin passes largely intact through the stomach and intestines. Along the way, it grabs hair and carries it out of the body, says H. Ellen Whiteley, D.V.M., a veterinary consultant in Guadalupita, New Mexico, and consultant for *The Country Vet's Home Remedies for Cats*. Give small pets between ½ and 1 teaspoon of canned pumpkin with every meal. Medium-size and large dogs can have between 1 teaspoon and 2 tablespoons of pumpkin with meals.

An alternative is to mix into their food flaxseeds or psyllium husks, which are available in natural food stores, says Joanne Stefanatos, D.V.M., a holistic veterinarian in private practice in Las Vegas. They act as natural laxatives, which help stools—and hair—move through the system more quickly. Give small pets about ¼ teaspoon of flaxseeds or psyllium with every meal. Larger dogs can take up to 1 tablespoon, she says.

Speed it through the system with a natural laxative. Combine raw oatmeal, honey, and olive oil into a paste and offer 1 to 2 tablespoons as a treat when hair balls are

Call the Vet

Sometimes hair balls get so large that they can't move in either direction—downward through the intestines or upward onto the carpet. These large masses of fur, called bezoars, can form hard-to-budge—and life-threatening—blockages.

"If your pet's stomach swells and he frequently vomits or can't pass his stool, see a veterinarian right away," says H. Ellen Whiteley, D.V.M., a veterinary consultant in Guadalupita, New Mexico, and consultant for *The Country Vet's Home Remedies for Cats.*

a problem, says Kathleen Carson, D.V.M., a holistic veterinarian in private practice in Hermosa Beach, California. For pets that experience hair balls regularly, you can give the mixture two or three times a week.

Giving pets ½ teaspoon of olive or safflower oil twice a day will have a similar effect, adds Dr. Stefanatos.

Reduce the discomfort. Hair balls can irritate the stomach and intestines, causing constipation or an upset stomach, says Dr. Carson. "Slippery elm bark (*Ulmus rubra*) can be really helpful," she says. She recommends diluting 20 drops of slippery elm tincture in an ounce of spring water and giving your pet one dropperful three times every day—20 minutes before morning and evening meals and again at bedtime. It is best to use tinctures that are alcohol-free because alcohol may be harmful for cats.

Groom away the problem. The most effective way to prevent hair balls, especially in cats, is to brush your pet every day. This removes loose fur before your pet has a chance to swallow it, says Dr. Carson.

Hives

The Signs
- Your pet has red welts and is unusually itchy.
- The skin on her face is swelling.

When dogs and cats brush against something that they are allergic to, they may break out in hives—ugly, itchy welts that can appear within minutes. Hives usually go away within 24 hours, but they sometimes come right back.

Mainstream veterinarians sometimes give pets antihistamines to quell the allergic reaction and, in severe cases, steroids to control inflammation. Since hives go away fairly quickly, it usually isn't necessary to use powerful drugs, says Stephanie Chalmers, D.V.M., a veterinary dermatologist and holistic veterinarian in private practice in Santa Rosa, California. A better approach is to use natural remedies to ease the discomfort—and to figure out why your pet is having reactions in the first place.

The Solutions

Give an oatmeal bath. To ease the itching of hives, Dr. Chalmers recommends filling the bathtub with cool water and adding half a packet of colloidal oatmeal (like Aveeno). Encourage your pet to soak in the water for about 10 minutes. If the water doesn't cover the itchy areas, pour water over his body until his fur and skin are soaked. Keep giving baths once a day until he feels better.

An alternative is a colloidal oatmeal compress. "Mix some oatmeal powder with cool water in a bowl until you get a milky solution. Then saturate a washcloth in the mixture, squeeze it out, and gently hold it over the irritated skin for 5 to 10 minutes," Dr. Chalmers advises.

Lather up some relief. Pet stores sell oatmeal shampoos, which can help relieve itchy skin. Dr. Chalmers recommends one that also contains aloe vera, a soothing herb. After working up a lather, let it soak into the fur for a few minutes, then rinse your pet well, she advises.

Brew some tea. Black and green teas contain tannins, which can help stop itching, says Dr. Chalmers. Brew some tea, allow it to cool, and pour it into bathwater. Or you can soak a cloth in room-temperature tea and apply it as a compress.

Soothe with flower essences. These essences can relieve itchy skin. A good combination is agrimony, beech,

Call the Vet

If hives keep coming back, it may mean your pet has a weak or damaged immune system. Sometimes hives are the first sign of a more serious allergic reaction. If your pet breaks out in hives and seems weak or is having trouble breathing, get him to a vet right away.

cherry plum, crab apple, olive, and walnut, says Wanda Vockeroth, D.V.M., a holistic veterinarian in private practice in Calgary, Alberta. Put 2 or 3 drops of each essence in a 1-ounce dropper bottle filled with spring or purified water. Give your pet a dropperful of the mixture twice a day. "You can also put it in a spray bottle and spritz the itchy spots or dab some on a cloth and wipe it on," she adds.

Beat the bees. For hives caused by insect stings, ease the discomfort with homeopathic Ledum or Urtica urens, says Dr. Chalmers. She recommends 30C potency, giving cats one to three pellets and dogs three to five pellets once a day. If necessary, repeat the treatment 24 hours later, she says. Use these remedies one at a time. If your pet doesn't improve in 2 to 3 hours, try another remedy.

Block the poison. Some dogs and cats are sensitive to poison ivy and break out in hives at the slightest contact. Homeopathic Rhus tox., given every 15 to 30 minutes for up to 2 hours, will often ease the discomfort, says Jeanne Olson, D.V.M., a holistic veterinarian in private practice in North Pole, Alaska. She recommends the 30C or 30X potencies. Pets under 50 pounds can take one pellet. Dogs 50 pounds and over can take two or three pellets.

Hot Spots

The Signs

- Your dog has one or more circular sores that are red, swollen, and oozing.
- The sores get larger within hours.
- The sores are painful, smelly, and hot to the touch.

During the warm months especially, the combination of bug bites, allergy flare-ups, and even matted hair can make dogs perpetually itchy. They react by scratching and biting their skin—sometimes for hours. "Eventually, all that scratching does damage," states Lowell Ackerman, D.V.M., a veterinary dermatologist in Mesa, Arizona, and author of the *Guide to Skin and Haircoat Problems in Dogs*.

Once the skin is damaged, bacteria move in and quickly spread among the hair follicles. This can cause painful, rapidly spreading sores known as hot spots. Cats rarely get hot spots, but they are quite common in dogs, especially breeds like Chow Chows, which have heavy double coats that often get matted. The sores can appear anywhere but usually crop up in areas dogs are able to reach, like on the tail, flanks, back, and rump.

Hot spots look scary, but in most cases they involve only the top layer of skin. You don't need to use powerful drugs or lotions, says Dr. Ackerman. Most hot spots are easy to treat with natural home remedies. Here is what veterinarians advise.

The Solutions

Dry the sores with Burow's. Available in some drugstores and grocery stores, this solution dries the sores and helps them heal more quickly, says Dr. Ackerman. He recommends spraying the hot spots with Burow's solution two or three times a day until they heal.

Coat them with boric acid. This natural element acts as a mild antiseptic and speeds healing, says Steven A. Melman, V.M.D., a veterinarian in private practice in Potomac, Maryland, and Palm Springs, California, and author of *Skin Diseases of Dogs and Cats*. He recommends dabbing a solution containing acetic and boric acids (like DermaPet Ear and Skin Cleanser), available from veterinarians, on hot spots once or twice a day.

Soothe pain with calendula (*Calendula officinalis*). Made from marigolds, calendula tincture helps ease the pain of hot spots, says Michelle Tilghman, D.V.M., a holistic veterinarian in private practice in Stone Mountain, Georgia. Dilute the tincture half-and-half with water and place the bottle in steaming (not boiling) water for 7 minutes to remove the alcohol. Apply it with a cotton ball two or three times a day.

Cool the heat with witch hazel. Hot spots can be warm to the touch. Cool things down with witch hazel. Apply

Call the Vet

These sores look ugly but are rarely serious. "They heal so quickly that you almost never need to give your dog antibiotics," says Lowell Ackerman, D.V.M., a veterinary dermatologist in Mesa, Arizona, and author of the *Guide to Skin and Haircoat Problems in Dogs*.

Sometimes, however, hot spots get so sore and tender that your dog won't let you near them. Less often, the infection that is causing the sore travels deep inside, rather than spreading across the surface of the skin. This usually occurs when the hot spot has been covered by a thick ointment, Dr. Ackerman explains.

Hot spots that are extremely tender or don't get better within a day or two need to be treated by your vet. He may need to give the sores a deep cleaning and possibly use medications such as steroids to reduce the inflammation.

with a cotton ball. It evaporates almost instantly, making hot spots feel more comfortable. You can use witch hazel two or three times a day, says Dr. Ackerman.

Brew some tea. Black tea contains tannic acid, which dries the sores and helps them heal more quickly, says Dr. Ackerman. Soak a tea bag in hot water, let it cool, and apply the bag directly to the sore for 5 minutes. Do this three or four times a day.

Stop the itch cycle. To stop the itching that causes hot spots, try a homeopathic remedy, such as HomeoPet Hot Spot Dermatitis, says Carolyn Blakey, D.V.M., a holistic veterinarian in private practice in Richmond, Indiana. Dogs can take 10 drops and cats 3 drops, both three times a day. If the problem doesn't go away in a few days or if it clears up and then returns, call your vet, she adds.

Stop the scratching from the inside out. Holistic veterinarians sometimes give dogs with hot spots a Chinese medicine called Armadillo Counter-Poison Pill. It contains a combination of herbs that can help relieve itchy skin. "I use it in place of antihistamines," says Dr. Tilghman. You can find Armadillo Counter-Poison Pill in health food stores and natural apothecaries. Give pets weighing under 15 pounds one pill a day. Pets 15 to 50 pounds can take two pills a day, and larger dogs can take three pills a day, she advises.

Stop the fleas. Hot spots often occur when dogs have an allergic reaction to flea bites, so it is essential to get rid of fleas as well as ticks, says Alexander Werner, V.M.D., a veterinary dermatologist in private practice in Studio City, California.

Comb out the mats. Hair mats that lie against the skin are another common cause of hot spots. "They are a great hiding place for fleas and ticks," says Dr. Ackerman. "And when moisture and heat collect, bacteria can grow like crazy."

Hair mats can be difficult (and painful) to remove because they lie so close to the skin. Preventing them is easy,

Give Them Air

Hot spots heal quickly as long as they get plenty of air and stay dry and clean. To help air circulate, use electric clippers or a pair of blunt-nosed scissors to trim a 1-inch border around the hot spot so that the fur is about ⅛ inch high.

Rinse the area thoroughly with warm water. Using a cotton ball, dab the spot with witch hazel, then gently pat it dry.

however. Just brush your dog at least twice a week, preferably once each day. Regular grooming also helps the skin breathe, which makes it harder for infections to get started, says Dr. Ackerman.

Discourage the licking. Saliva helps some wounds heal—but dogs can take a good thing a little too far. They sometimes lick hot spots so long and so vigorously that they never heal. Try distraction instead, says Susan G. Wynn, D.V.M., a veterinarian in Atlanta and coeditor of *Complementary and Alternative Veterinary Medicine*. A treat or a walk around the block can help your dog focus on something other than the hot spot. A game of catch or a quick training session can also help.

Insect Bites and Stings

The Signs
- Your pet has one or more raised, itchy bumps on her skin.
- The area around the sting is red and swollen.

Most stings aren't too serious, but even small amounts of toxin can raise a painful, itchy bump. Veterinarians often recommend treating stings by applying hydrocortisone ointment, which reduces inflammation. Although hydrocortisone is safe for pets, many veterinarians prefer a more natural approach.

The Solutions
Remove the stinger. "If the stinger stays in your pet's skin, there will be a stronger reaction and more likelihood of an allergic response," says Nancy Brandt, D.V.M., a holistic veterinarian in private practice in Las Vegas. To

The Healing Instinct

When dogs and cats get stung or bitten by insects, their immediate response is to start licking. A wet tongue is more than just soothing. "The enzymes in saliva help to neutralize poisons," says Patricia Cooper, D.V.M., a holistic veterinarian in private practice in Houston. When they are bitten in a place where they can't lick, they will often rub the area on grass or in the dirt in an attempt to eliminate the venom, she adds.

remove the stinger, put your fingers at the base of the bump and squeeze upward. This will push the stinger up so that it is easier to remove with your fingers or tweezers. Don't push down on the bump, or you will push more of the venom into the skin, she says.

Apply a mud poultice. Mud acts like a sponge and pulls venom out of a sting. It also helps reduce inflammation, says Beatrice Ehrsam, D.V.M., a holistic veterinarian in private practice in New Paltz, New York. You can leave the mud on the sting until it dries out, she adds.

Apply chamomile tea. Reduce the irritation by soaking a cotton ball or a piece of gauze in room-temperature chamomile tea and applying it to the sting, says Dr. Brandt. Leave the compress in place for 15 to 30 minutes and repeat three times on the first day. For the next 2 days, apply a fresh compress for a few minutes three times a day.

Cover it with a tea bag. Black tea contains compounds that help draw toxins out of a sting, says Mona Boudreaux, D.V.M., a holistic veterinarian in private practice in Albuquerque, New Mexico. Moisten a tea bag in warm water, squeeze it out, and then hold it on the sting for 10 to 15 minutes, she advises.

Treat it with Ledum. This homeopathic remedy helps puncture wounds heal and prevents swelling as long as you give it quickly after the sting occurs, says Patricia Cooper, D.V.M., a holistic veterinarian in private practice in Houston. She recommends giving two or three tablets of Ledum 30C, either by putting them in your pet's mouth or by dissolving them in a few teaspoons of water and then putting the water in your pet's mouth. Repeat the treatment every 30 minutes for 2 to 3 hours, she advises.

Ease the irritation. For small bites from gnats, the essential oils lavender and thyme quickly relieve irritation and itching, says Dr. Brandt. Mix 3 drops of either oil in a teaspoon of apple cider vinegar and dab the solution on the bites, she advises. Vinegar by itself is also effective.

Apply some ammonia. It's another way to ease the pain, says Susan G. Wynn, D.V.M., a veterinarian in Atlanta and coeditor of *Complementary and Alternative Veterinary Medicine*. A number of commercial products, like After Bite, use ammonia as the active ingredient.

Give an oatmeal bath. Sometimes pets—usually puppies or kittens—lie down on a pile of ants and wind up with a rash of itchy bites on their bellies. Stop the itching fast by soaking them in cool water spiked with oatmeal, says Dr. Boudreaux. Put about a cup of oatmeal in a cloth and tie it up with a piece of string. Put the bag in a cool-water bath and soak your pet for about 20 minutes. You can repeat the treatment once a day until the rash and itching improve, she says.

Reduce inflammation with an Indian herb. The herbal supplement ashwagandha (*Withania somnifera*), available in health food stores, reduces inflammation caused by stings, says Tejinder Sodhi, D.V.M., a holistic veterinarian in private practice in Bellevue and Lynnwood, Washington. You can add ashwagandha powder to your pet's food. Pets under 15 pounds can take ¼ teaspoon of the powder two or three times a day. Those weighing 15 to 50

Call the Vet

For pets with allergies, a single sting can be deadly. "If your pet has an allergic reaction, with severe swelling around his head or neck, difficulty breathing, persistent pain, or drowsiness, go to the vet right away," says Beatrice Ehrsam, D.V.M., a holistic veterinarian in private practice in New Paltz, New York. He may need a shot of epinephrine, a medication that blocks a serious allergic reaction called anaphylaxis. You should also call your vet if your dog or cat has been bitten by a black widow or a brown recluse spider.

If you can't get to a vet immediately, try the homeopathic remedy Apis, giving two or three 200C pills, says Gerald Buchoff, B.V.Sc.A.H. (bachelor of veterinary science and animal husbandry, the Indian equivalent of D.V.M.), a holistic veterinarian in private practice in North Bergen, New Jersey. "It works immediately," he says. Apis will help get your pet past the danger, but you will still have to get him to a vet as quickly as possible, he says.

pounds can take ½ teaspoon two or three times a day, and dogs over 50 pounds can take as much as 1 teaspoon two or three times a day.

Stop swelling with spice. Another Indian remedy for inflammation is the spice turmeric (*Curcuma longa*). Dr. Sodhi recommends mixing powdered turmeric with a little chicken broth and slipping it in your pet's food. "It's bland, despite its bright yellow color," he adds. Pets under 15 pounds can take about ½ teaspoon of turmeric twice a day. Those that weigh 15 to 50 pounds can take 1 teaspoon twice a day, and larger pets can have 2 teaspoons twice a day.

Itching

The Signs

- Your pet scratches or bites his skin.
- His coat looks patchy.
- The skin is raw and inflamed.
- He chews on his paws.
- He scratches his ears or shakes his head.

Itching is usually caused by allergies to pollen, molds, fleas, or even food. It's most likely to be a problem when your pet's overall health isn't what it should be, says Jordan A. Kocen, D.V.M., a holistic veterinarian in private practice in Springfield, Virginia.

Mainstream veterinarians usually treat the itching itself by giving antihistamines, for example, while holistic vets focus more on the underlying problems, which can range from emotional stress to problems with the immune system. Here is what holistic veterinarians recommend.

The Solutions

Stop fleas with neem. This Indian herb (*Azadiracta indica*) repels fleas and soothes sore skin, says Michael W. Lemmon, D.V.M., a holistic veterinarian in Renton, Washington, and past president of the American Holistic Veterinary Medical Association. Neem can be applied to the skin as an oil or lotion. One popular brand available from veterinarians is PhytoGel, which contains neem along with other essential oils. Neem has a bitter taste that fleas dislike. Dogs and cats dislike it, too, which means they are less inclined to bite and chew at their skin, he says.

Neem is also available in capsule form, Dr. Lemmon adds. Ask your vet what dose is right for your pet.

Cool the skin. The herb calendula (*Calendula officinalis*), also known as marigold flowers, soothes hot, irritated areas on your pet's skin, says Charles E. Loops, D.V.M., a veterinarian in private practice in Pittsboro, North Carolina. He recommends adding 10 to 15 drops of calendula tincture to 4 ounces of distilled or spring water and putting the mixture in a spray bottle. Spray the area as often as needed to help stop your pet from scratching. It is best to use tinctures that are alcohol-free because alcohol may be harmful for cats.

The herbs chickweed (*Stelleria media*) and plantain (*Plantago*, various species) are also good for skin problems, says Dr. Lemmon. You can buy both herbs as a lotion, or you can use bulk leaves to brew a tea. Boil a pint of water and pour it over 2 tablespoons of dried herbs or a handful of fresh herbs. Cover and steep for 10 to 20 minutes. Let cool to room temperature, strain, dip a cloth in the solution, and apply it to your pet's sore spots for 5 to 10 minutes a few times a day.

Give him extra zinc. Research has shown that zinc supplements can help relieve a variety of skin problems, including itching. Veterinarians usually recommend chelated zinc. Ask your vet what dose is right for your pet.

Give him extra fatty acids. Two common fatty acids, omega-3s and omega-6s, can help reduce itching and inflammation, says Susan G. Wynn, D.V.M., a veterinarian in Atlanta and coeditor of *Complementary and Alternative Veterinary Medicine*. You can buy supplements that contain both of these fatty acids in health food and pet supply stores. Ask your vet which supplement and dose are right for your pet.

Slip some vegetables into his bowl. Increase the amounts of immunity-boosting nutrients in your pet's diet with raw vegetables like carrots and green beans, Dr. Kocen says. If your pet doesn't like raw vegetables, chop and lightly steam them, then mix them in his food.

Give him vitamin supplements. The vitamins A, C, and E have been shown to strengthen the immune system and may help reduce itching, Dr. Lemmon says.

- Vitamin A helps irritated skin heal and strengthens the immune system. This nutrient can be harmful in large amounts, however, so check with your vet for the correct dose.
- Vitamin C strengthens the immune system and may help relieve allergies. Give cats and dogs weighing under 15 pounds 250 milligrams of vitamin C a day. Pets 15 to 50 pounds can take 500 milligrams, and larger dogs can take 1,000 milligrams. Vitamin C may cause diarrhea, so experiment with the dose until you find an amount your pet will tolerate.
- Vitamin E reduces inflammation in the skin and is essential for healthy immunity. Give cats and dogs under 15 pounds 100 international units (IU) of vitamin E a day. Dogs 15 to 40 pounds can take 200 IU. Those 41 to 70 pounds can have 400 IU, and dogs over 70 pounds can take 800 IU, says Dr. Lemmon.

Stop itching with homeopathy. Holistic veterinarians often treat itchy pets with homeopathic Sulfur, Petroleum, or Graphites, Dr. Lemmon says. Each of the remedies can be effective, but pets react to them differently, so check with your vet before using them at home, he adds.

Soothe him with an oatmeal bath. A classic remedy for itchy skin is to lather pets with an oatmeal shampoo or to soak them in cool water to which you have added colloidal oatmeal (like Aveeno), says Dr. Loops. Many vets prefer colloidal oatmeal to shampoo because it doesn't contain soaps that may irritate itchy skin. Give your pet a bath every day for 2 or 3 days. After that, if it doesn't seem to be working, find another way to soothe the skin.

Kennel Cough

The Sign
- Your dog has a dry, hacking or gagging cough.

Kennel cough is caused by different viral and bacterial infections that spread from dog to dog, usually in kennels, says Allen M. Schoen, D.V.M., director of the Veterinary Institute for Therapeutic Alternatives in Sherman, Connecticut, and author of Love, Miracles, and Animal Healing.

Kennel cough may be treated with antibiotics or cough suppressants, and mainstream vets often recommend vaccinations to prevent it. These are pretty serious treatments for a condition that usually goes away on its own in a few weeks, says Adriana Sagrera, D.V.M., a holistic veterinarian in private practice in New Orleans. Veterinarians who practice alternative medicine usually favor a drug-free strategy for keeping kennel cough under control. Here is what they advise.

The Solutions

Stop it with loquat. This Chinese herbal liquid soothes your dog's irritated throat, says Dr. Schoen. He recommends giving dogs under 15 pounds ⅛ teaspoon of loquat a day. Dogs 15 to 50 pounds can take ½ teaspoon, and larger dogs can take ½ to ¾ tablespoon. You can get loquat from mail-order companies.

Since loquat is very sweet, Dr. Schoen adds, don't give it to dogs that have diabetes without first checking with your veterinarian.

Battle the infection. The herbs echinacea (*Echinacea purpurea* or *Echinacea angustifolia*) and goldenseal (*Hydrastis canadensis*) have antiviral and antibacterial properties, says Dr. Schoen. He recommends giving dogs with kennel cough an extract that combines both of these herbs. Dogs under 15 pounds can take 7 drops twice a day, and larger dogs can take 15 drops twice a day. The taste is very bitter, he adds, so disguise the drops by mixing them in your dog's food.

Use a natural cough syrup. Homeopathic remedies for kennel cough are available as a soothing syrup, says Christina Chambreau, D.V.M., a holistic veterinarian in Sparks, Maryland, and education chairperson for the Academy of Veterinary Homeopathy. Two popular brands

Harness That Cough

Dogs with kennel cough go into a coughing frenzy at the slightest pressure from a collar and leash. While your dog recovers, it is a good idea to swap his usual collar for a harness that buckles around the chest. This will keep him under control without putting pressure where it hurts.

Questionable Protection

Many kennels recommend that dogs be vaccinated against kennel cough before being boarded. But some vets specializing in natural healing feel the vaccinations may cause problems.

"Vaccinations can compromise the immune system and weaken an animal overall," says Christina Chambreau, D.V.M., a holistic veterinarian in Sparks, Maryland, and education chairperson for the Academy of Veterinary Homeopathy. "Giving repeated vaccinations for diseases that aren't life-threatening is not good for the health of the animal."

The problem is that without the vaccination you may have trouble finding a kennel that will board him. Or you may be asked to sign a release saying that you won't hold the owners responsible should your dog get infected.

If you get your dog vaccinated, keep in mind that the shot provides protection for less than 6 months.

are Hyland's Cough Syrup and B and T Homeopathic Cough and Bronchial Syrup.

"Some dogs lick the syrup, but for others, you will need to squirt it down their throats with a needleless syringe," she says. She recommends giving dogs under 15 pounds one-quarter of the human dose. Dogs 15 to 50 pounds can take one-half of the human dose, and larger dogs can take the full human dose.

Try lemon and honey. Dr. Chambreau recommends mixing 2 tablespoons of honey and a teaspoon of lemon juice in ½ cup of water and giving the solution to your dog a few times a day.

Ease congestion with mullein. The herb mullein (*Verbascum thapsus*), available in capsule form, is very effective at breaking up the congestion that often accompanies kennel cough, says Beatrice Ehrsam, D.V.M., a holistic veterinarian in private practice in New Paltz, New York. "You can empty the capsule into hot water to make a tea, then cool it down and squirt it in his mouth with a needless syringe," she says. Or you can empty the capsule into his food. She recommends giving mullein twice a day until your dog's cough is getting better. Give dogs under 15 pounds one-quarter of the human dose. Dogs 15 to 35 pounds can take one-half of the human dose, and dogs 36 to 60 pounds can take three-quarters of the human dose. Larger dogs can take the full dose.

Help the body heal itself. The vitamins E, C, and A strengthen the immune system and can help dogs with kennel cough heal more quickly, says Dr. Ehrsam. Dogs under 15 pounds can take 30 to 100 international units (IU) of vitamin E, 250 to 500 milligrams of vitamin C, and 500 IU of vitamin A a day. Dogs 15 to 40 pounds can take 200 to 300 IU of vitamin E, 500 milligrams of vitamin C, and 1,000 IU of vitamin A a day. Larger dogs can take 400 IU of vitamin E, up to 1,000 milligrams of vitamin C, and 5,000 IU of vitamin A a day. Since vitamin C can cause diarrhea, you may have to cut back the dose until you find an amount your pet will tolerate.

Mange

The Signs

- Your pet scratches furiously.
- Her skin looks red and irritated, or there are bumps or sores.
- She is losing patches of hair or has a bad smell.

Any dog can get it, and sometimes cats get it, too.
There are two kinds of mange. One kind, called scabies, occurs when sarcoptic mites tunnel under the skin and trigger an allergic reaction. Scabies is highly contagious to pets as well as people, which is why it is important to treat all the pets in your family even when only one is infected, says Susan G. Wynn, D.V.M., a veterinarian in Atlanta and coeditor of *Complementary and Alternative Veterinary Medicine*.

The second kind of mange, called demodectic mange, occurs when demodex mites, which normally live on the skin, suddenly multiply to enormous numbers. Demodectic mange usually occurs in puppies because their immune systems are changing constantly and aren't able to control the mites, says Dr. Wynn.

Both types of mange can cause ferocious itching, which is why holistic and mainstream veterinarians sometimes recommend killing the mites quickly with a medication called ivermectin (Stromectol). Other vets use a toxic dip. But drugs may not be necessary as long as you keep your pet's natural immunity strong and use home remedies to control the itching, says Jane Laura Doyle, D.V.M., a holistic veterinarian in private practice in Berkeley Springs, West Virginia.

The Solutions

Kill mites with a natural dip. A quick way to eliminate mange mites is to douse your pet with a lime-sulfur solution, says Steven A. Melman, V.M.D., a veterinarian with practices in Potomac, Maryland, and Palm Springs, California, and author of *Skin Diseases of Dogs and Cats*. Available from vets, products such as Lymdyp are safe and very effective, although you will probably have to repeat the treatment about once a week until your pet is feeling better.

Soothe the skin with an oatmeal bath. "Shampoos containing oatmeal can help in relieving the itch caused by mange," says Dr. Doyle. Be sure to use an oatmeal shampoo made specifically for pets, she adds. Human shampoos may be harmful for dogs and cats.

Use natural medicines to strengthen immunity. Holistic veterinarians sometimes recommend giving pets reishi mushroom (*Ganoderma lucidum*) supplements, available in pet supply and health food stores, says Dr. Wynn. She recommends giving pets under 20 pounds one-quarter of the human dose. Those weighing 20 to 50 pounds can take

Call the Vet

Sometimes a small patch of mange spreads to other parts of the body. This can be serious, if only because it usually occurs when another, underlying problem—like genetic immune deficiency, a hormonal imbalance, diabetes, or cancer—has weakened the immune system and allowed the mites to thrive.

It is fine to treat small patches of mange at home, but call your vet if it seems to be spreading.

half the human dose. Dogs 51 to 80 pounds can take three-quarters of the human dose, and larger dogs can take the full human dose.

Another herb that strengthens immunity is astragalus (*Astragalus membranaceus*), which is given in the same amounts as reishi mushrooms. Charlene Kickbush, D.V.M., a dog breeder and holistic veterinarian in private practice in Watkinsville, Georgia, advises giving astragalus along with echinacea (*Echinacea angustifolia* or *Echinacea purpurea*). The dosage recommendations for astragalus and echinacea are the same as those given previously for reishi mushroom.

Give a vitamin supplement. Nutrients such as vitamins C and E help strengthen immunity and block the release of histamine, a chemical in the body that causes itching, says Nancy Scanlan, D.V.M., a holistic veterinarian in private practice in Sherman Oaks, California. Pets under 15 pounds can be given about 100 international units (IU) of vitamin E a day, along with 250 milligrams of vitamin C. Those weighing 15 to 40 pounds can take 200 IU of vitamin E and between 500 and 1,000 milligrams of vitamin C. Dogs 41 to 80 pounds can take 400 IU of vitamin E and

1,000 milligrams of vitamin C, and dogs over 80 pounds can take 600 IU of vitamin E and between 1,000 and 2,000 milligrams of vitamin C. Every pet needs different amounts of these nutrients, so ask your vet for the precise dose.

Keep things calm. Pets with demodectic mange tend to have flare-ups whenever they are stressed. Do everything you can to keep your pet calm and comfortable until the mange clears up, says Dr. Kickbush.

Give the house a thorough cleaning. The mites that cause scabies can survive for several days even when they are off your pet. To prevent a reinfestation, vacuum rugs, sweep and mop floors, and wash your pet's bedding, crate, collar, and any grooming tools that you happen to use.

Overweight

The Signs
- Your cat has a potbelly.
- Your dog doesn't have a waist.
- You can't feel your pet's ribs.
- He snores or is having trouble breathing.

About one in three pets in this country is overweight. Blame it on a combination of overeating and under-exercising.

Traditionally, veterinarians have recommended "light" diets to take off the pounds. But low-calorie foods don't work for all pets. And because these foods are low in certain fatty acids, they can cause dry, flaky skin and a dull coat, says Susan G. Wynn, D.V.M., a veterinarian in Atlanta and coeditor of *Complementary and Alternative Veterinary Medicine*. Another problem is that low-calorie diets are typically very low in fat, so some pets become intolerant to fat in the future. This means that they could develop pancreatitis if they are ever switched back to a regular food, she says.

Here is what holistic veterinarians advise for permanent girth control.

The Solutions

Try a fat-burning herb. Holistic veterinarians sometimes recommend a Chinese herbal formula called Coptis Purge, which helps the body burn more fat, says Ihor Basko, D.V.M., a holistic veterinarian in private practice in Honolulu and Kilauea, Hawaii. You have to give Coptis Purge for only 3 to 5 days. "It doesn't take much to work really well," he says. You can buy Coptis Purge in health food stores. Every pet will need a different amount, so check with your vet before giving it at home, he advises.

Another herb that can reduce body fat is hawthorn berry (*Crataegus laevigata*). It improves liver function, which helps reduce the amounts of fat and cholesterol in the blood, says Dr. Basko. He recommends 10 milligrams of hawthorn berry three times a day for every 10 pounds of weight. Hawthorn berry can be dangerous for pets with heart disease, however.

Switch to a natural diet. Most commercial pet foods contain way too much fat and not enough fiber, says Dr. Basko. They are also highly flavored, so dogs and cats tend to eat more than they really need. Switch to an all-natural pet food that more closely duplicates the balance of nutrients that nature intended. You can buy natural foods such as Innova, PetGuard Premium, Wysong, and Solid Gold in some pet supply stores and from mail-order companies.

A homemade diet may be even better, say holistic veterinarians. For cats, the diet should be 50 to 60 percent raw meat, 20 to 30 percent grains, such as rice or millet,

Call the Vet

Cats that don't eat for a day or two have a high risk of developing fatty liver disease, or hepatic lipidosis. Going without food may prompt body fat to migrate into the liver, overloading it, and possibly shutting it down. There is nothing wrong with reducing the number of calories your cat consumes or giving him a different food, adds Anne Lampru, D.V.M., a holistic veterinarian in private practice in Tampa, Florida. Just make the change slowly because cats sometimes refuse to eat when the menu changes. If your cat does stop eating, don't wait more than a day or two before calling your vet, she says.

with the rest coming from cooked vegetables. For dogs, the diet should be 35 percent protein from meat, 30 percent grains, and 35 percent raw or cooked vegetables. To kill harmful organisms such as salmonella, you can lightly steam meat before adding it to your pet's food. Your vet may also advise giving your pet nutritional supplements.

Make the change gradually by mixing the new and old foods together, gradually increasing the percentage of new food over a few weeks, says Anne Lampru, D.V.M., a holistic veterinarian in private practice in Tampa, Florida. Dogs adjust fairly quickly, but cats may take as long as a month before they are entirely comfortable with the new diet, she says.

Control the food flow. Many overweight pets have food available all the time. This is convenient for owners, but it makes it easy for pets to overindulge. A better strategy is to feed your pet twice a day, once in the morning and again in the afternoon, says Dr. Wynn.

Round out his meals with vegetables. Try giving your pet about 25 percent less of his regular food and replacing it with chopped raw or cooked vegetables, says Donn W. Griffith, D.V.M., a holistic veterinarian in private practice in Dublin, Ohio. (Don't use onions, which can be dangerous for cats.)

Vegetables have fewer calories than grains or meats, says Dr. Wynn. And because they are high in fiber, your pet will feel full even when he is getting fewer calories.

If your pet hasn't lost any weight in 4 weeks, reduce the pet food by another 25 percent. If you still don't see any changes, talk to your vet about finding a more efficient weight-loss plan, says Dr. Wynn.

Stimulate his metabolism with massage. Giving your pet a vigorous whole-body rubdown stimulates everything from digestion to circulation to the activity of the adrenal glands. The faster your pet's "motor" runs, the more calories he will burn, says Dr. Basko, who recommends giving overweight pets a 20- to 30-minute massage once a day.

Rebalance his body with glandular supplements. Some pets gain weight after being spayed or neutered because the hormonal balance affecting metabolism has been altered, says Dr. Lampru. You can help restore your pet's normal metabolism by giving him glandular supplements, available in health food stores. Cats and dogs weighing less than 15 pounds can take about one-sixth of the human dose once a day. Pets between 15 and 50 pounds can take one-third of the human dose, and dogs over 50 pounds can have about one-half of the human dose, she says.

Burn off fat with exercise. Start with 5 minutes of exercise three to five times a week, then, as your pet can tolerate it, increase the duration to 20 to 60 minutes a day, says Dr. Wynn. Too much exercise can be harmful for pets that are elderly or have heart problems, so talk to your vet before starting an exercise routine.

Entertain their brains along with their stomachs. Many dogs and cats depend on food to keep them entertained, says Dr. Lampru. Keep their minds busy with interactive toys such as the Buster Cube or the Goody Ship. Although toys like the Buster Cube use food to get pets' attention, they aren't able to eat much, and the fun of trying to get it out keeps them entertained for hours.

Get cats moving with catnip. "If they are really lethargic, you may have to get them stimulated with catnip first," says Dr. Basko. Catnip, both fresh and dried, lowers their inhibitions, he explains. "They will be more willing to play games and exercise," he says. Give cats ¼ to ½ teaspoon of dried catnip, recommends Dr. Wynn.

Pad Cracks

The Signs
- Your pet's paw pads are rough, crusty, cracked, or swollen.
- She limps on one or more paws.

The paw pads are shock-absorbing cushions covered with thick, durable skin. They can easily withstand the wear and tear of normal ramblings. But when the skin on the pads cracks or bleeds, walking becomes painful. Cats occasionally have pad cracks, but they are much more likely to occur in dogs.

Veterinarians usually treat cracked paw pads with lotions or oils, and that is the best way to help them heal. But treating the cracks doesn't go far enough, says Donna M. Starita, D.V.M., a holistic veterinarian in private practice in Boring, Oregon. Here are a few ways to treat and prevent pad cracks, starting on the inside and working your way out.

The Solutions

Heal them with minerals. "Many of the cracked pads I see are caused by a zinc or selenium deficiency in the diet," says Dr. Starita. Zinc strengthens the skin and helps it heal more quickly, while selenium boosts immunity so that the body is better able to heal itself. She recommends giving pets weighing under 30 pounds 2.5 to 5 milligrams of zinc and 50 micrograms of selenium a day. Larger pets can take 5 to 10 milligrams of zinc and 100 micrograms of selenium a day. You can give your pet these supplements for 2 weeks at a time.

Speed healing with vitamin E. This nutrient improves blood circulation so cracked pads heal more quickly, says Dr. Starita. It also strengthens immunity and helps prevent parasites or infections from causing cracking. You can give pets under 15 pounds 50 international units (IU) of vitamin E a day. Those weighing 15 to 50 pounds can take 100 IU, and larger dogs can have 200 IU of vitamin E a day. She recommends opening a vitamin E gel capsule and squeezing the oil into your pet's food.

Soften the pads with oil. You don't want to moisturize the paw pads too much because they need to be tough to maintain their strength. But when the pads are cracked, applying a little sesame or olive oil will help them heal, and the oils are safe if your pet decides to lick them off, says Kathleen Carson, D.V.M., a holistic veterinarian in private practice in Hermosa Beach, California.

Lotions containing vitamin E are also good, although you will need to keep your pet distracted for a few minutes while the lotion soaks into the skin. It is best to use all-natural lotions, available at health food stores.

Increase internal moisture. Dogs and cats with internal problems like infections can lose tremendous amounts of water from their bodies, causing the pads to crack, says

George Carley, D.V.M., a holistic veterinarian in private practice in Tulsa, Oklahoma. Chinese medicines containing rehmannia root can strengthen the organs and help prevent moisture loss, he says.

Rehmannia root is used in many different formulas, he adds. When cracked pads are caused by kidney problems, for example, your vet may recommend using Rehmannia 6. If lung problems are to blame, your pet may need Rehmannia Schizandra Formula. Check with a veterinarian who practices traditional Chinese medicine to get the right formula and dose for your pet.

Strengthen the skin with fatty acids. Fatty acids build and maintain the membranes of skin cells as well as reduce inflammation that may accompany pad cracks. Dr. Starita recommends giving pets a fatty-acid supplement called Eskimo Oil, available from veterinarians or in drugstores. Pets love the taste, so you can put it in their mouths or mix it in their food. Cats and dogs under 15 pounds can take ⅛ teaspoon of Eskimo Oil twice a day. Pets weighing 15 to 50 pounds can take ¼ teaspoon twice a day, and larger dogs can take ½ teaspoon twice a day.

Stop infections with pau d'arco. This herb (*Tabebuia impetiginosa*) contains a natural substance called quechua that kills fungi, bacteria, and some viruses, says Joanne Stefanatos, D.V.M., a holistic veterinarian in private practice in Las Vegas. She recommends combining equal parts pau d'arco tincture and mineral oil and applying this mixture to the pads once a day until the cracks start to heal.

Ringworm

The Signs
- Your pet has bald patches that are spreading.
- The fur breaks off close to the skin.
- He has crusty or scaly sores.

Ringworm is a fungus that makes itself at home in the outer layers of the skin, nails, and hair. It is not uncommon for healthy cats to carry around the fungus and not get symptoms as long as their immune systems keep it in check. (Dogs with ringworm invariably have symptoms.) When ringworm temporarily gets the upper hand, however, it gives off toxins that can damage the skin and hair, causing bald patches on the head, paws, or back.

Ringworm is highly contagious, both to pets and people, so it is important to call your vet when you suspect that your pet is infected, says Robert Kennis, D.V.M., a veterinary dermatologist at Texas A&M University College of Veterinary Medicine in College Station. More common in cats than dogs, ringworm usually isn't serious, although it may spread over the entire body and cause crusty sores.

The traditional treatment for ringworm is to give an oral drug such as griseofulvin. The medication is very effective, but it may cause dangerous side effects, says Dr. Kennis. Most holistic veterinarians feel that it is better to soothe the discomfort and fight the ringworm naturally until it goes away on its own. Here is what they advise.

The Solutions

Soothe the sores. The herb calendula (*Calendula officinalis*) relieves inflammation and can help ringworm sores heal more quickly, says Michelle Tilghman, D.V.M., a holistic veterinarian in private practice in Stone Mountain, Georgia. She recommends applying calendula tincture to the sores, using a cotton swab, every day until they heal. Or apply goldenseal (*Hydrastis canadensis*) tincture to the sores two or three times a day, using a cotton ball. It is best to use tinctures that are alcohol-free because alcohol may be harmful for cats.

Wash away fungal food. Dousing your pet with apple cider vinegar will clear away skin cells that are ringworm's main source of nourishment, says Joanne Stefanatos, D.V.M., a holistic veterinarian in private practice in Las Vegas. A vinegar rinse (2 tablespoons of apple cider vinegar in 1 quart of water) helps relieve itching as well. Repeat once a week, after shampooing, as needed.

An alternative is MalAcetic shampoo, available from veterinarians. It contains vinegar and other ringworm-fighting ingredients, says Steven A. Melman, V.M.D., a veterinarian with practices in Potomac, Maryland, and Palm Springs, California, and author of *Skin Diseases of Dogs and Cats*.

A Glowing Diagnosis

Ringworm resembles many other skin problems, such as allergies, mange, and skin infections. So veterinarians developed a special test for it: They turn out the lights.

When patches of ringworm damage are illuminated with a type of black light (called a Wood's lamp) in a dark room, they sometimes glow in the dark, says Robert Kennis, D.V.M., a veterinary dermatologist at Texas A&M University College of Veterinary Medicine in College Station.

The light works on only certain strains of ringworm, he adds, so some pets may be infected even when they don't have the glow.

Bleach it away. Ringworm spores can survive anywhere in the house and are capable of reinfecting pets for up to a year after they have been treated. To get rid of the spores, Dr. Kennis recommends wiping counters, floors, and other areas in the house with household bleach. Straight bleach is best, although you can dilute 1 part bleach in 10 parts water when you are washing delicate surfaces like linoleum or wood.

Keep him confined. Until he's completely healed, confine your pet to one area in the house, says Dr. Kennis. This will make it easier to control and eliminate ringworm spores that are constantly drifting off his coat. Some veterinarians recommend keeping pets in a stainless steel cage until the ringworm is gone, although keeping them in a small room with a tile floor that is easily cleaned also helps contain the fungus.

Clean the carpets. Vacuum the house every day to pick up contaminated hairs and spores; remove the vacuum bag and seal it inside a plastic garbage bag. "You can also steam-clean carpets, upholstery, drapes, and the like," says

Alexander Werner, V.M.D., a veterinary dermatologist in private practice in Studio City, California.

Update your pet's wardrobe. When pets with ringworm start scratching, the spores go flying. Dressing your pet in an old T-shirt and putting socks on his feet will help control the fungus and prevent him from nibbling and scratching the sore spots, says Dr. Stefanatos. Washing the clothes in bleach and drying them thoroughly can also be helpful because the bleach will kill the spores. "It can decrease itchiness by 50 percent or more," she says.

Protect yourself. The ringworm fungus is contagious, so don't handle your pet too much until he has recovered. Dr. Kennis advises wearing a smock when you are treating the sores or even cuddling your pet. Afterward, wash your hands thoroughly with bleach, followed by a rinsing with hot, soapy water. Pets with ringworm should always be kept away from young children or people who are already ill because they are more vulnerable to the fungus than those whose immune systems are strong.

Treat all your pets. Ringworm is readily passed from pet to pet. Treat even those that aren't yet infected, says Dr. Melman. If you don't, the spores are sure to survive and cause trouble all over again.

Give extra support. Some cats have weakened immune systems that allow ringworm to hang on even when they are getting medical treatment. Reishi mushroom (*Ganoderma lucidum*) and astragalus (*Astragalus membranaceus*), taken together, strengthen the immune system and help cats with chronic ringworm battle the infection while they are taking medication, says Susan G. Wynn, a veterinarian in Atlanta and coeditor of *Complementary and Alternative Veterinary Medicine*. She recommends giving 3 drops of each tincture once a day, either by mixing the tinctures in broth or butter or by adding them to your cat's food.

Ticks

The Signs
- You keep finding tick "balloons" on your pet.
- Your pet has suddenly lost his appetite.

Although ticks are ugly to behold, their bites usually aren't painful and don't cause itching. But they can transmit serious diseases like Rocky Mountain spotted fever and Lyme disease, so it is worth doing everything you can to keep them away. This is especially important for dogs because they get ticks much more often than cats. "Cats are very sensitive to things on their coats and usually get rid of ticks quickly by licking or scratching them off," says Lori Tapp, D.V.M., a holistic veterinarian in private practice in Asheville, North Carolina.

To keep the critters away, mainstream veterinarians sometimes recommend using tick collars or, more recently, medications that can be applied to the coat or taken orally. Even though the medications are usually safe, they are essentially pesticides that stay in (or on) your pet's body for a long time. Most holistic veterinarians favor a more natural approach that helps strengthen his natural defenses, making ticks less likely to cause diseases, says Christina Chambreau, D.V.M., a holistic veterinarian in Sparks, Maryland, and education chairperson for the Academy of Veterinary Homeopathy.

The Solutions

Boost immunity with echinacea. Pets are much less likely to get infected with tick-borne illnesses when their immune systems are working well. The herb echinacea (*Echinacea purpurea* or *Echinacea angustifolia*) has been shown to strengthen the immune system, says Michele Yasson, D.V.M., a holistic veterinarian in private practice in New York City and Rosendale, New York. "Use one-quarter of the recommended human dose for cats and dogs that weigh less than 20 pounds." Pets 20 to 50 pounds can take one-half of the human dose, and dogs over 50 pounds can take the full human dose. You can give echinacea for about 2 weeks at a time.

The easiest way to give echinacea is to open the capsules and sprinkle the powder in your pet's food. When using liquid echinacea, put a few drops in water and mix the solution in the food, she advises. Don't use liquid echinacea that contains alcohol because pets dislike the taste, she adds.

Repel ticks with essential oils. "The combination of cedarwood and citronella essential oils seems to be an effective tick repellent," says Jeffrey Levy, D.V.M., a holistic veterinarian in private practice in Williamsburg, Massachusetts. He recommends mixing equal amounts of the two oils together and diluting them with rubbing al-

Call the Vet

The tick that causes Lyme disease is much smaller than the usual "dog ticks." Many dogs get infected and their owners never even see the culprit. That is why it is essential to recognize the signs of tick-borne infections.

"If your dog's appetite falls off and he gets listless and lethargic, or if you notice he has pain, swelling, or heat in any of the joints, take him to a vet as soon as possible," says Lori Tapp, D.V.M., a holistic veterinarian in private practice in Asheville, North Carolina. Other warning signs of tick infections include diarrhea, vomiting, limping, or difficulty breathing.

Also call your vet when you know your pet has been bitten by a tick, even if he seems fine. Illnesses caused by ticks are much easier to treat when you catch them early, says Dr. Tapp.

cohol, using 1 part oil to 10 parts alcohol. Shake the mixture and apply a small amount to your pet's lower legs before he goes outside. Some pets will insist on licking the oils off, in which case you should try another remedy instead.

Even though it is safe to apply diluted essential oils externally, they may interfere with some homeopathic treatments, Dr. Levy adds. "If your pet is getting homeopathy, check with your vet before using the oils."

Keep them away with garlic. Garlic contains compounds that are secreted through the skin, and ticks and fleas find it distasteful, says Dr. Tapp.

She recommends giving your pet fresh raw garlic (powdered doesn't work) every day. Cats can have about ⅛ teaspoon of fresh garlic a day for no more than 2 weeks since too much garlic can cause a certain type of anemia. Dogs over 50 pounds can have as much as 2 teaspoons a day, and smaller dogs can have ¼ to ½ teaspoon. Most dogs like the taste, so you can just stir some in their food, says Dr. Tapp.

Check for ticks often. It takes ticks quite a bit of time to penetrate the skin and start feeding, and a lot longer—more than 24 hours in some cases—before they can transmit diseases. When you pick ticks off your pet within a few hours after they climbed on, they are unlikely to be a problem. "You can often find ticks by feeling your pet well with your hands or using a flea comb," says Dr. Yasson. Flea combs are small-toothed combs that readily pick up even small ticks. She recommends doing a tick patrol at least once a day during the warm months, especially when your pet has been spending time outside.

Remove the critters. It is best to use tweezers, although you can remove ticks with your fingers as long as you wear gloves or grip the tick with a small piece of plastic wrap. "Grab the tick as close to the skin as possible, then pull gently and slowly," says Dr. Levy. Don't twist them out. In most cases, the head will pull out of the skin, and you can discard the tick in a small jar of rubbing alcohol. Don't worry if the head stays in the skin, he adds. It will fall out on its own over time.

Soothe the wound. You might see a bump or some redness on your pet's skin afterward. "Apply a natural herbal salve such as a comfrey ointment to the tick bite," says Dr. Yasson.

Or apply a little tea tree oil, adds Beatrice Ehrsam, D.V.M., a holistic veterinarian in private practice in New Paltz, New York. "It's a good antiseptic. Dilute a few drops in 1 ounce of water and apply it with a cotton ball." Don't let your pet lick the area until the salve has soaked into the skin. (Avoid using tea tree oil on cats because it can be dangerous to them.)

Clear the underbrush. Ticks thrive in many parts of the country, and you will never get rid of them all. Ticks live a foot or two off the ground in scrub and grasses, Dr. Tapp explains. "Keep your pet from running in areas where ticks tend to frequent, and get rid of underbrush and low branches in your yard." It is also a good idea to keep your grass mowed short. Pets that play on well-mowed lawns are much less likely to get ticks, she says.

Vomiting

The Signs
- Your pet is retching.
- You're finding messes on the floor.

Dogs and cats throw up all the time, whether they're sick or not. And they barely seem to notice. But their people worry about it. The advice from vets is simple: As long as the vomiting is sporadic and the pets seem chipper and don't have diarrhea, it probably doesn't mean much of anything.

The usual reasons for vomiting are they ate tainted food, they're feeling stressed, or they ate too much too fast, says Holly Cheever, D.V.M., a veterinarian in Guilderland, New York. Vomiting that lasts more than a day needs to be checked by a vet, but here's how to avoid garden-variety throwing up.

The Solutions
Feed them more often. People customarily feed their dogs once a day because it's convenient and the dogs don't

complain. But the hungrier dogs are when breakfast rolls around, the faster they're going to eat. Dr. Cheever recommends feeding them at least twice a day, and three or four times is probably better. Don't increase the total amount they eat, she adds. Just spread out the servings so that pets don't overwhelm their stomachs by stuffing it in.

Be consistent. Dogs are surprisingly sensitive to changes in their diets. Switching to a different brand of food, or even a different flavor of the same brand, will often make them sick for a day or two. Dogs don't need variety in their diets. If you do change foods, make the change slowly by mixing in a little bit of the new food with a lot of the old, then adding a greater proportion of the new stuff every day. After about 5 days, they'll be ready to make the change entirely and probably won't get sick, says Richard Levine, V.M.D., a veterinarian in Toms River, New Jersey.

Deal with the hair-ball issue. Cats often vomit because the hair they ingest during grooming isn't digested. When it forms an uncomfortable wad, problems occur. Cats often improve when they switch to a food that's high in dietary fiber—one that contains between 3.5 and 10 percent fiber. "I like Vetasyl, which comes as a gelatin capsule filled with powdered fiber," says Jane Brunt, D.V.M., a veterinarian in Towson, Maryland. Available from veterinarians, Vetasyl helps keep the stomach full and calm and helps hair balls move through the system more quickly.

Dab petroleum jelly on the roof of the mouth. Cats don't like the taste, but putting a dab of petroleum jelly on the roof of their mouths every few days lubricates the digestive tract and helps swallowed hairs pass smoothly through, rather than jamming up in the stomach. Since putting your finger in a cat's mouth isn't always the safest move, vets sometimes recommend putting the petroleum jelly—or a commercial hair-ball remedy—under the nose. Cats don't like the taste, but they like the sticky sensation even less and will lick it off, says Karen L. Campbell, D.V.M., professor of dermatology and endocrinology at the University of Illinois College of Veterinary Medicine at Urbana–Champaign.

Brush the heck out of them. Cats are always shedding, and brushing them once a day will remove loose hairs before they get swallowed, says J. M. Tibbs, D.V.M., a veterinarian in District Heights, Maryland. You can follow this up by giving them a wipe with a moist washcloth, which will remove even more loose hairs.

Worms

The Signs

- Your pet vomits or has diarrhea.
- He scoots his bottom across the floor.
- There are small fragments or whole worms in the stool.
- He is thin, though he eats well.
- He seems tired.

Many puppies and kittens are born with intestinal worms or get them soon after birth. Adult pets also get worms, which cause symptoms ranging from diarrhea to an itchy bottom.

Many types of worms don't cause serious problems, but they should still be taken seriously because pets tend to get worms when their immune systems aren't as strong as they should be, says Michele Yasson, D.V.M., a holistic veterinarian in private practice in New York City and Rosendale, New York.

Pets with worms are usually given oral medications. The medications, available over the counter and from

Know What to Look For

Tapeworms don't cause obvious physical symptoms, but you can often see the ricelike worm segments around your pet's rear end or in his stool.

Roundworms may cause vomiting, diarrhea, a pot-belly, or a dull coat. Look for beige, spaghetti-like worms in the stool, especially in puppies and kittens.

vets, are very effective, but you don't want to use them again and again, says Christina Chambreau, D.V.M., a holistic veterinarian in Sparks, Maryland, and education chairperson for the Academy of Veterinary Homeopathy. That is why holistic veterinarians prefer to use a preventive approach. A stronger and healthier pet is much less likely to get worms in the first place.

The Solutions

Add bran to his diet. One way to get worms out of the intestinal tract is to give your pet oat or wheat bran, says Dr. Chambreau. She recommends adding a little bit of bran—½ teaspoon for cats and dogs under 15 pounds and 2 teaspoons for larger pets—to their regular food every day.

Eliminate worms with herbs. An herbal combination called Para-L, sold as a liquid, helps remove worms from the body, says Dr. Chambreau. Ask your vet how much to give and the best way to use it safely.

Add garlic to his food. This pungent herb helps clean and "tonify" the intestines, possibly killing some of the worms, says Dr. Chambreau. Dogs over 50 pounds can have as much as 2 teaspoons of garlic a day, and smaller dogs can have ¼ to ½ teaspoon a day. Cats shouldn't be given more than ⅛ teaspoon of garlic a day for about 2 weeks. You can chop or mince the garlic and add it directly to your pet's food. Or you can puree it in a little water, along with some fresh vegetables.

Give him sweet potatoes. Pets with worms sometimes have digestive troubles such as diarrhea. A tasty way to soothe their stomachs is with sweet potatoes, says Beatrice Ehrsam, D.V.M., a holistic veterinarian in private practice in New Paltz, New York. "Give your pet cooked sweet potatoes every day," she suggests. Pets under 15 pounds can have 2 teaspoons of sweet potatoes a day, and larger pets can have 1 tablespoon or more, she says.

Put some spice in his food. Cayenne pepper and hot-pepper sauces such as Tabasco create an inhospitable environment in the intestines, and some worms may simply

Call the Vet

Some types of worms, such as tapeworms, are visible in the stool, but others stay out of sight, in the intestines, quietly removing blood and essential nutrients. As the worm population increases, your pet may get increasingly tired and weak. He may be vomiting and have diarrhea, and his belly may be distended as well.

Worms pose another danger: Children who play in areas where infected dogs have been may get infected themselves.

Worms sometimes go undetected because the symptoms can be caused by a variety of problems. It is worth asking your vet to check for worms during your pet's annual checkup. (Be sure to bring along a fresh stool sample, which is used to detect worms.) In the meantime, if your pet suddenly seems tired and lethargic and he doesn't get better within a few days, make an appointment to see your vet.

pack up and leave, says Dr. Chambreau. "Start with a few drops or sprinkles and increase the amount until your pet lets you know he doesn't like it anymore. Then back off."

Put him on a rich diet. Worms that live in the intestines can rob your pet of essential nutrients. To keep him well-nourished while he is being treated, give him a diet that is high in both protein and fat, says Lori Tapp, D.V.M., a holistic veterinarian in private practice in Asheville, North Carolina. For dogs with worms, about 40 percent of the diet should come from meat or eggs; for cats, protein should make up 60 percent or more of the diet. To increase the amount of fat in the diet, you can add a little butter or canola or olive oil to his food, she says. Or you can temporarily switch your pet to puppy or kitten food, which is much richer than foods that are made for adults. If your pet is sensitive to changes in his diet, however, or has had pancreatitis in the past, it is best not to change his diet even temporarily.

Increase the iron with raw liver. Some intestinal parasites remove large amounts of blood from the intestines, causing a drop in iron. Giving your pet raw organic liver once a day for 2 to 4 weeks will quickly restore the iron that is lost, says Dr. Tapp. "Liver should make up no more than 15 percent of the meat in his diet."

Improve digestion with enzymes. To help your pet get the most nutrition from his food, give him digestive enzymes, such as Prozyme, says Dr. Ehrsam. You can give ¼ teaspoon of the enzyme for every cup of food. Keep giving the enzyme until your pet is free of worms, she advises.

Another way to maximize nutrition is to give your pet acidophilus, which contains beneficial bacteria that improve digestion, says Dr. Ehrsam. She recommends giving one capsule twice a day to dogs weighing 15 pounds or more and half a capsule twice a day to smaller pets.

PART THREE

Common Behavior Problems

Barking and Meowing

Most dogs don't need an excuse to bark. Voices in the yard next door will get them started. So will the arrival of the mail carrier or the sound of sprinklers. Or they'll bark just to pass the time.

Cats are less likely to indulge in aimless noisemaking, but they can be very persistent when they want something. And some breeds, such as Siamese, are much more "talkative" than others.

No one objects to occasional barks and meows. But when it happens too much and too loudly, there are problems, says Larry Lachman, Ph.D., an animal-behavior consultant in Carmel, California, and author of *Dogs on the Couch* and *Cats on the Counter*.

Pets that are always making noise are trying to tell you something, and they aren't going to quit until you resolve whatever it is that's bothering them, says John C. Wright, Ph.D., a certified applied animal behaviorist; professor of psychology at Mercer University in Macon, Georgia; and author of *The Dog Who Would Be King* and *Is Your Cat Crazy?* "You need to understand their emotions and motivations in order to correct the noisemaking."

Most noisy pets are looking for extra attention, he explains. And they aren't shy about demanding it. They'll keep barking or meowing until you stop whatever it is you're doing in order to attend to them. Food won't keep them quiet, at least not for long. And they don't really want to go outside. They want to be catered to, and they'll keep asking for attention until they feel satisfied.

It's never easy to know for sure what's causing dogs to bark or cats to meow, adds Liz Palika, a trainer in Oceanside, California. She recommends keeping a journal for a few weeks in which you write down everything that's happening when your pet starts making noise. By putting together various clues—the time of day, who was home and who was gone, whether there were noises outside, and what sorts of activities were going on—you'll eventually see a pattern that will help you determine what's triggering the outbursts.

Once you know what's causing barking or meowing, you can move on to the next step, making it stop. Here's what the experts advise.

The Solutions

Ignore the noise. Yelling "Quiet!" rarely stops pets from barking or meowing. For one thing, they don't know what the word means. More important, they interpret your yelling as participation, and that can really get the calland-response going.

"Whenever you look at, speak to, pet, or otherwise reward dogs and cats, you're reinforcing what they're doing at the moment," says Dr. Lachman. "It's important not to engage in these or other types of rewarding behaviors while your pet is vocalizing."

You can take the cold-shoulder treatment one step further by leaving the room whenever your pet starts making noise. Since barking and meowing are usually bids for at-

The Direct Approach

It doesn't help to punish dogs for barking, but trainers sometimes recommend looking them in the eye, holding their mouths closed for a second or two, and telling them no. The combination of eye contact and a stern command puts them on notice that you're in charge and that they need to pay attention. And because dogs dislike having their mouths held closed, they'll begin to associate barking with this unpleasant sensation and will look for other ways to get your attention.

tention, turning your back and walking away give a powerful signal. Dogs and cats are observant and resourceful, and when they realize that making noise isn't getting their message across, they'll do it less often.

Keep them occupied. Dogs and cats tend to make the most noise when they're bored and full of energy, says Kimberly Barry, Ph.D., a certified applied animal behaviorist in Austin, Texas. "Giving them something else to do can really help," she says. Take them for a walk or play in the yard. Toss them a ball. Busy pets are usually quiet pets, and once they blow off steam, they'll be less likely to bark or meow later on.

Block stimulating sounds. Dogs' hearing is vastly superior to ours. This means they can hear—and respond to—things that we're not even aware of, from rustling in the bushes to the sound of a mouse in the ceiling. Increasing the level of background noise by turning on the radio, TV, or a fan helps mask many of the noises that cause dogs to bark, says Dr. Wright.

Reduce their anxiety. It doesn't happen very often with cats, but some dogs get so lonely and anxious when they're alone that they bark frantically. Their anxiety doesn't start when you shut the door, Dr. Wright adds. They usually start getting nervous when you're doing all the little things that indicate you're about to leave, like picking up your keys or putting on your coat.

You can reduce their overall anxiety by making these predeparture signals a little less meaningful with sheer repetition, says Dr. Wright. On a day you're going to be home, for example, pick up your keys and rattle them as though you're going to leave—then sit back down. A minute later, rattle them again. Do this periodically all day long. Put on your coat and take it off. Open and close the garage door. Walk out the door and quickly walk back in. The idea is to strip away the concept of "leaving" from all these little gestures. After a while, your dog will understand that the rattle of keys doesn't mean very much, so his anxiety won't reach such a fever pitch when you're ready to go out the door.

Begging

When your pet's ancestors wanted something, they either had to be tough enough to take it or quick enough to grab it without getting caught. Begging was out of the question.

Things changed when dogs and cats became domesticated. "Pets beg from humans because humans control their resources," says Kimberly Barry, Ph.D., a certified applied animal behaviorist in Austin, Texas.

Some begging isn't a problem, Dr. Barry adds. Cats that meow when their food is being poured, or dogs that stare hungrily when they're waiting for supper, aren't being unusually pushy. But some pets never take no for an answer. And unless you teach your pets that begging isn't appreciated, they'll continue to cross the line.

Anyone who lives with an attention hog or a food mooch soon discovers that giving in "just this once" never stops begging. Once pets learn that they can get the goods by demanding them, they're not about to be patient. They're going to either get what they want or drive you crazy until you deliver.

Begging won't be an issue if you never give in to your pet's demands, Dr. Barry says. But once dogs and cats start the habit, you'll need to be more creative in finding ways to make them stop. Try these vet-approved tactics.

The Solutions

Satisfy them with service. It may seem as though pets have insatiable appetites—for food or whatever else they desire—but they do have a satisfaction "ceiling," a point at which they've essentially had enough. You can help pets reach this ceiling by giving them what they want on a regular, predictable schedule, says Dr. Barry. Give them their food at the same times every day. Take a few extra minutes to play with them or take them for walks. Go out of your way to give them attention, rather than wait for them to come to you. Once they understand that all things come to those that wait, they'll naturally get a little less demanding, she explains.

Be strong and ignore them. It's not the easiest solution, but the most effective way to stop begging is to make it unprofitable by never giving in. The drawback to this approach is that you'll have to live with a lot of meowing, nudging, or whining in the meantime. Pets that are used to getting what they want can be extremely demanding and persistent, and bad habits don't go away in a day or two, says Dr. Barry. You may have to put up with the begging for a few weeks or even months. It's worth gritting your teeth and going through with it, she advises.

Cure them with kindness. It's nearly impossible to share a kitchen or dining room with a mooching dog without scolding him, and even St. Francis would have yelled "Quiet!" after 20 minutes of feed-me-now meows. But venting your natural feelings will intensify their efforts because pets that are begging are looking for attention, and scolding and yelling are just other forms of attention, Dr. Barry says.

Rather than scold pets when they beg, praise them when they don't, she advises. Suppose you're working in the kitchen and your dog happens to be staying out of your way and minding his own business. Go over and pet him. Dogs and cats crave our approval, and experts have found that praising good behavior usually works better than punishing rudeness.

Be consistent. Dogs and cats are a lot like children. Even when they understand what they should and shouldn't do, they're always willing to push their advantage. No matter how strict you are most of the time, giving in teaches them that begging does pay off as long as they do it long enough. "If you're not consistent, you're almost like a slot machine," says Robin Kovary, director of the American Dog Trainers Network in New York City. "They know that if they keep pulling the lever, eventually they'll hit the jackpot."

Chewing

All dogs like to chew, and the retriever breeds are especially fond of it, says Marty Becker, D.V.M., a veterinarian in Bonners Ferry, Idaho, and coauthor of *Chicken Soup for the Pet Lover's Soul*. His own Labrador, Sirloin, culminated his chewing career by gnawing the Christmas decorations—bulbs, extension cords, and all—from the outside of the Beckers' house.

Though retrievers are among the worst offenders, they hardly have the chewing market cornered. Dogs use their teeth to express their feelings. They chew when they're happy or sad. They chew when they're bored. And sometimes they chew just because it feels good to do it.

Cats have their own forms of vandalism, but they're rarely chewers, adds Robin Downing, D.V.M., a veterinarian in Windsor, Colorado. "Cats tend to be destructive with their claws," she says.

A puppy's urge to chew peaks between 14 and 24 weeks. That's when they are teething, and chewing helps ease their aching gums, explains Dr. Downing. Most dogs outgrow the urge to chew. But some dogs continue to be oral throughout their lives. Some of the reasons include the following.

- *Boredom.* Grown dogs that do a lot of chewing are usually bored, says Inger Martens, a trainer and behavior consultant in Los Angeles. Chewing is one way dogs burn off energy that they're not releasing in other ways, she explains.
- *Anxiety.* Chewing is a way for some dogs to release negative feelings and console themselves, says Dr. Becker.
- *Habit.* Dogs may chew on sofas or socks simply because no one ever taught them not to.

The Solutions

Since dogs chew as naturally as they breathe, it would be impossible—and cruel—to make them stop. Yet you don't want to sacrifice your personal belongings to your dog's voracious pleasures. The solution is to compromise: Encourage dogs to chew, but make sure they understand what constitutes an appropriate chew toy. As long as you're consistent and vigilant for a few weeks, most dogs learn pretty quickly to distinguish a soggy tennis ball from your favorite shoes. Here's a plan that trainers recommend.

Give him something else to chew. Pet supply stores are packed with chew toys, ranging from rubber balls and nylon bones to pig ears. Dogs have preferences, so you may have to experiment until you find the one your dog likes best, Dr. Downing says. Shop for texture and consistency; most dogs like toys that provide a little *al dente* resistance. A universal favorite happens to be the cheapest: Nearly every dog adores used tennis balls, and you can usually find a few in the grass or bushes surrounding neighborhood courts.

"Mark" the toys. Since dogs are intensely attracted to odors, new toys don't always generate a lot of excitement. Dogs chew your possessions largely because they have your scent, so it's a good idea to rub new toys between your palms for a while, says Dr. Downing.

Reward him. As soon as your dog starts chewing an authorized toy, show some excitement, suggests Dr. Downing. Praise and play with him. Throw the toy so he can grab it and bring it back. He'll discover that this particular toy has lots of potential, and he'll keep returning to it to repeat the fun. At this point the toy is truly his, and you're ready for the next step: Teaching him what he can't chew.

Stay alert. The first weeks of a stop-chewing program are the toughest because you're trying to break old habits—or prevent new habits from taking hold. Once dogs get the opportunity to chew something they shouldn't, the pleasurable experience is something they'll remember. So you essentially have to act like a doggy cop, keeping your dog in sight all the time.

Bait and switch. When you catch him putting something verboten in his mouth, quickly take it away and replace it with his toy, praising him when he takes it, says Dr. Downing. When you're not around to supervise, keep him in an area where he doesn't have access to temptation. If you can deny him the opportunity for unsupervised chewing for a few weeks, you'll be able to reinforce the idea that his toys are acceptable for chewing, while *yours* are not.

Apply repellent. It's not uncommon for dogs to get fixated on particular objects, like shoes or chair legs. Since you can't supervise dogs all the time, apply a pet repellent to the target areas. Repellents such as Grannick's Bitter Apple spray or cream have a terrible taste, and most dogs will stay away from objects that have been treated. You don't have to use a repellent forever, Dr. Downing adds. Dogs learn from experience.

If the Bitter Apple or other repellents don't do the job, be prepared to experiment. Hot-pepper sauce can be a very effective deterrent, although you'll want to test it first to make sure it doesn't stain.

Keep him active. Dogs that don't get a lot of exercise and don't have a lot to do are the ones most likely to chew, so it's essential to help them burn off excess energy, Dr. Downing says. Chasing a ball or going for regular walks allows dogs to blow off steam. Active dogs get to be tired dogs, she adds. This means they'll be more likely to spend their time napping rather than chewing.

Fear of Noises

It's difficult to imagine life as dogs hear it. Their hearing is about four times better than ours. Many experts believe that dogs have a nearly instinctive fear of loud noises, such as thunder during a storm or the sonic boom of a jet or the bang of a firecracker.

"To top it off, they usually have something bad happen to them during a thunderstorm, like getting stuck under the bed or knocking over furniture while trying to hide," says Katherine Houpt, V.M.D., Ph.D., a board-certified veterinary behaviorist, professor of physiology, and director of the behavior clinic at Cornell University College of Veterinary Medicine in Ithaca, New York. "The whole experience can be quite devastating." Their frantic behavior during storms, she explains, is really just a cry for help.

Cats don't love loud noises and are sometimes skittish about gunshots or sudden claps of thunder, but it's mainly dogs that suffer—and that show their fears by shaking, shivering, or trying to hide, says Dr. Houpt. "Dogs' ears are more sensitive to those low, deep frequencies than cats' ears are. And though small dog breeds certainly can be afraid during storms, it's more common in larger dogs because they often hear those frequencies best."

The fear of loud noises is among the more stubborn behavior problems that veterinarians treat. With a little work and patience, however, nearly every dog can learn to tolerate, if not appreciate, loud noises. Here's what the experts recommend.

The Solutions

Create a safety zone. In their evolutionary pasts, dogs were den-dwelling animals, and they're still attracted to small, enclosed spaces, especially when they're frightened. "They like having confined quarters where they can feel sheltered from the elements," says D. Caroline Coile, Ph.D., a researcher specializing in canine senses, who raises and shows salukis near Tallahassee, Florida. "They can become particularly stressed when they feel exposed and vulnerable."

Dogs that are afraid of loud noises will invariably gravitate toward the smallest, coziest hiding place they can find—under beds, in the backs of closets, or in some cases even in bathtubs. You can help them feel more secure by creating special hiding places that they can consider their own, Dr. Coile advises. "Try putting a dog bed in some nook or cranny of the house, like beneath the stairs or behind a chair, where the dog can feel protected. That may be all she needs."

Take away the fear. Dogs don't process their memories and experiences as well as people do, which means their ninth thunderstorm or Fourth of July is just as scary and unexpected as the first. Since they won't learn from experience, it's up to their people to change the pets' thinking so that loud noises don't frighten them anymore. Behaviorists deal with noise anxiety by using a technique called systematic desensitization. Put more simply, it means getting them used to noise, says Dr. Houpt.

The principles of desensitization therapy are complex, and there are many ways to go about it. The basic technique, however, is simple. Here's how it works.

- Gradually and gently expose your dog to very low levels of whatever it is she fears. For example, buy a recording of a thunderstorm and play it for about 15 minutes at a very low volume, says Dr. Houpt. At first the volume should be so low that your dog doesn't show any sign of fear. Every 5 minutes or so, give her a treat or praise as a way of rewarding her for being calm. This will help her understand that the sound she's hearing is a predictor of something good rather than something scary.

- On the second or third day, increase the volume just slightly until your dog starts looking a little bit uneasy. As long as she stays calm, give her praise and treats. You may want to do some basic obedience drills as well. This will help distract her from the noise and help her understand that good behavior is always rewarded, whether there's noise in the background or not.

- With daily practice, most dogs will start getting less fearful. They'll be able to tolerate louder volumes without getting frightened, and they'll be able to listen to the recordings for longer periods of time. What they'll discover is that loud noises—thunderstorms, fireworks, or anything else—really aren't such a big deal.

When you are doing desensitization therapy, you don't want to crank up the volume too high or too fast, says Dr.

Houpt. Rather than help your dog accept the noise, this will scare her half to death, she explains. Going slowly—for some dogs, it takes months to overcome their fears—is the best way to ensure success.

Reward calm behavior, not the fears. Act as though there's nothing to be afraid of. It's natural to want to reassure a dog that's trying to crawl behind a bookcase, but this tends to make the fear worse, says Alex Brooks, director of Alex Brooks School of Dog Training in Des Plaines, Illinois. "Though you don't want to treat a scared pet harshly, you don't want to coddle her too much either," he explains. "She'll learn not only that it's okay to be scared but also that being scared has its rewards."

Dogs always take their cues from their owners, he adds. When you act calm and relaxed, dogs will naturally be a little less frightened. At the same time, you need to help them understand that only good behavior gets rewards, never fearful behavior. So when your dog starts getting nervous, tell her to sit and stay, Brooks suggests. "Then praise her and reward her for being so good and sitting still. Repeat this every time there's a storm or other noises, and your dog will learn that she'll be rewarded if she sits and stays by your side."

Play in the rain. The fear of thunderstorms is probably the most common fear that behaviorists deal with. Dogs will never like loud noises, but you can teach them that thunderstorms can be fun in other ways. "I act as though it is just like any other afternoon and encourage the dogs to come out and play with me," Brooks says. "I praise them generously for fetching balls and romping around. Every time a storm starts brewing, I take them out and play for a few minutes again. Eventually, they learn through repetition that storms mean good times."

The problem with this is that most dogs are afraid not of rain but of thunder, and when there's thunder, there's

sure to be lightning. Make sure that there's safe shelter before going out in the elements, he advises.

Ask your vet about medications. Most dogs can learn to
tolerate loud noises, but some are so terrified that nothing
seems to help. These dogs often improve when they're
given sedatives or anti-anxiety medications such as fluoxetine (Prozac). Sometimes the drugs are used to help dogs
get through difficult periods, such as Fourth of July week-
ends. More often, they're used in combination with a desensitization program. "They can help dogs get through
drastic situations until the behavior-modification training
takes hold," says Dr. Coile.

House Soiling

House soiling is one of the most frustrating and destructive of all behavior problems. Over time, it can lead to permanent odors or damage. Worse, it can cause a growing distrust between pets and their people.

Except for puppies (and sometimes kittens) that haven't yet learned to control their bodily functions, house soiling is rarely an accident. Pets that suddenly start making messes are trying to tell you something with their actions that they can't say in words. The message could be as simple as "I'm lonely" or "The litter box is a mess, and I'm not using it until it's clean."

"Yelling isn't going to help," says Gwen Bohnenkamp, owner of Perfect Paws, a dog and cat training center in the San Francisco Bay area, and author of *From the Cat's Point of View*. "You're not communicating anything to your pet except that you're really mad. And she probably won't have the slightest clue why."

Dogs view the house as their den. It's the place where they eat, sleep, and play. They don't want to make messes there. Many house cats take a slightly different view. Because the house is their whole world, they learn to associate different rooms with different activities. The kitchen is the place to eat. And the bathroom is the place to go to the bathroom (unless you put the litter box somewhere else).

Once dogs learn to do their business outside, they almost always continue to do so. Once cats accept a litter box as a suitable substitute for soft ground, you won't have too many surprises. But sometimes dogs and cats start going where they shouldn't. They're trying to tell you something. To find out what, start with the obvious explanations and solutions and work toward the more complicated ones.

The Solutions

Check the litter box. While some cats happily use the litter box even when it's been a few days since you changed the litter or cleaned out the clumps, others aren't so accommodating. "We flush a toilet every time we use it. Why should we expect a cat to accept a dirty toilet?" says Gregory Bogard, D.V.M., a veterinarian in Tomball, Texas. Litter boxes don't have to be pristine, but it's a good idea to clean out the box at least once a day. Then add a thin layer of new litter, Dr. Bogard suggests.

Check your schedule. For dogs, the most common cause of house soiling is a full bladder. Even though some dogs can last all day without a break, you really can't expect a dog to go for long stretches without occasionally having an accident. And once she's had an accident, she's much more likely to have another one because she'll come to associate the smell of the "spot"—or the entire room—with doing her business.

The solution is to let your dog out or walk her more frequently, says Dr. Bogard. People who work all day

Litter Box Basics

"Cats don't have accidents," says Gregory Bogard, D.V.M., a veterinarian in Tomball, Texas. "If they don't like the way the litter box is set up, they'll let you know." Here's how to avoid problems.

Supply enough boxes. The general rule is one box per cat, plus one. That means two boxes for one cat, three boxes for two cats, and so on, says Gwen Bohnenkamp, owner of Perfect Paws, a dog and cat training center in the San Francisco Bay area, and author of *From the Cat's Point of View* and *Manners for the Modern Dog*. This is especially important if your home has more than one floor or if you have a cat that tends to guard a box against use by another cat.

Forget the gizmos. Box lids, doors, and other fancy add-ons can distract or confuse your cat. "All your cat wants is a quiet, open box to do her business," says Bohnenkamp.

Keep it clean. Veterinarians recommend cleaning the box every time your cat uses it and adding about ½ inch of fresh litter over the top. Scented litter is okay as long as your cat doesn't mind, Dr. Bogard says. "Cats will use whatever litter you put down for them, but they're not fooled by a pretty scent. If the box is dirty, your cat knows."

Make it accessible. A cat can't use a litter box if the bathroom or closet door is closed. Make sure the box is in a place your cat can reach easily. If you have to move the box, do so a little bit at a time—no more than a foot a day. Moving a box too quickly can confuse and distract cats, and unanticipated messes may be the result, says Dr. Bogard.

often try to slip home at lunch. Or they hire a professional pet sitter to drop by once or twice a day. Vets often recommend training dogs to stay in a crate while you're out because dogs are extremely reluctant to eliminate in "their" space.

Check her health. It's not uncommon for dogs and cats to get bladder infections, kidney stones, or other conditions that can make it hard for them to control their bladders or bowels. When they start having accidents after years of good bathroom habits and you can't figure out why it's happening, you should consider the messes a valuable warning sign and call your vet right away.

Deal with fear and anxiety. Any change in routine can be very upsetting to pets. And they'll sometimes respond with unpredictable behavior. "It can take a while, from a few days to a few weeks or even more, for pets to get used to change," Dr. Bogard says. In the meantime, give them extra attention at every opportunity. The more time you're able to spend with your pet—with extra walks, for example, or additional strokes at bedtime—the less likely she'll be to express her insecurity in inappropriate places.

Set rules for the new house. Almost all pets are more prone to house soiling when they move to a new house, in part because they have to learn what rules apply to their new space. The best way to reduce the trauma of moving is to introduce your pet to one or two rooms at a time. Keep her in the bedroom for a few days, Bohnenkamp suggests. When she seems comfortable there, let her explore the upstairs for a while. Then give her the run of the downstairs. Moving slowly like this helps prevent pets from being overwhelmed with the change, she explains.

"Cats don't always like excessive freedom," Bohnenkamp adds. "Keeping them in one fairly large room with the litter box can help them explore slowly and ease their anxiety." If your cat has an accident after exploring the house, move her back into the first room and wait a few more days, he suggests.

It's a good idea to keep dogs in a room with a floor that can withstand a few accidents, says Bohnenkamp.

Stay low-key. Any intense emotion, like the excitement they feel when you come home from work, may cause some dogs to urinate on the spot, says Andy Bunn, a trainer in Charlotte, North Carolina. This so-called submissive urination doesn't occur in cats, he adds.

You can usually stop submissive urination by keeping your comings and goings low-key, Bunn says. When you walk in the door, don't look at, pet, or talk to your dog, he suggests. Just go about your business for a couple of minutes. Then ask your pet to sit, and greet her quietly. By that time, she'll be calm enough that she'll be less likely to lose control.

The same low-key approach works when you have guests in the house. As soon as they walk in the door, dis-

Urinating outside the Box

It's common for unneutered cats to urinate on walls or furniture as a way of defining their territory. (Accidents on the floor, on the other hand, are usually caused by other factors.) Females occasionally spray, but it's much more common in males.

The easiest way to stop this type of house soiling is to have your pet neutered, says Gregory Bogard, D.V.M., a veterinarian in Tomball, Texas. This causes a drop in male hormones, making spraying less likely. It's important to stop the problem early. Some pets that get into the habit of spraying keep it up even when they've been neutered, he adds.

tract your dog by having her sit or lie down or by playing with her for a few seconds. "Just give her something to think about other than the new people," Bunn says.

Be a little less "authoritative." Don't stand over your dog when giving her attention, and don't move your hands too quickly, Bunn adds. For a nervous dog, your looming body position is perceived as a show of dominance, and she may urinate in order to show she's subordinate to your authority.

Don't overreact. Anger—or, worse, punishment—doesn't stop house soiling. In fact, it can be counterproductive and will probably make your pet even more upset. "Your pet won't understand why you're yelling. If anything, scolding will teach her to be even more secretive about where she goes the next time," Dr. Bogard says.

Myths to the contrary, dogs and cats don't have accidents just to spite you. They're only trying to tell you that something is out of kilter, and they're confused and upset. So the best thing you can do is remain calm, says Dr. Bogard. Clean up the mess and use an odor remover to eliminate the scent. Then take a little time to figure out what's going wrong.

Act quickly. If you actually catch your pet in the act, try to distract her before she makes a mess by clapping your hands, for example. She'll probably stop what she's doing. That gives you the opportunity to gently take her where you want her to go—the litter box for cats and outside for dogs. When she resumes her business in the proper place, praise her in a low-key way and let her know what a good girl she is. You'll find that a little positive communication may be all it takes to get her back into the groove.

Jumping Up

One of the most common complaints among owners is that their dogs leap up whenever they or other people walk in the door, leaving paw prints behind or even knocking people over. It was once thought that dogs jumped up as a way of asserting dominance. Most animal behaviorists now believe that dogs jump up simply because they're excited to have company. (Although cats do their share of jumping—onto kitchen tables and windowsills—they rarely jump up on people.)

"Dogs have learned to be very face-oriented," explains Benjamin Hart, D.V.M., Ph.D., professor of physiology and behavior at the University of California, Davis, School of Veterinary Medicine and author of *The Perfect Puppy: How to Choose Your Dog by Its Behavior.* "They know that if they want to get petted or find out when they'll get their next meal, they need to have us look at them. They jump up to get our attention."

It's not always easy to teach dogs that jumping isn't the best way to get your attention. What you can do is to show them appropriate alternatives, praise them when they get it right, and consistently follow up bad behavior with consequences, says John C. Wright, Ph.D., a certified applied animal behaviorist; professor of psychology at Mercer University in Macon, Georgia; and author of *The Dog Who Would Be King* and *Is Your Cat Crazy?* "It's up to us to communicate in such a way that they understand what we want them to do or not to do." Here are a few tips you may want to try.

The Solutions

Turn a cold shoulder. Since dogs jump up because they want to be noticed, the best thing that you can do is to ignore them when their paws leave the ground, says Katherine Houpt, V.M.D., Ph.D., a board-certified veterinary behaviorist, professor of physiology, and director of the behavior clinic at Cornell University College of Veterinary Medicine in Ithaca, New York. "Your dog wants attention. If you start pushing him down or waving your hands around, that's exactly what he's getting," she explains.

Rather than push him away, turn away from him and fold your arms across your chest, she advises. "If you keep ignoring him, eventually he will learn that his jumping up isn't working, and he'll sit down. When he does, you can say hello and pet and praise him."

Tell them straight. Dogs look to us to tell them what is and isn't appropriate, and giving clear commands helps them understand what's expected, says canine researcher Marc Bekoff, Ph.D., professor of environmental, population, and organismic biology at the University of Colorado in Boulder. When your dog jumps up, hold out your hand in a "stop" gesture and forcefully tell him "Off," he suggests. Good behavior comes from clear communication, he explains. When your dog knows that you're displeased

Obedient Jumping

"Hearing dogs" are invaluable to those who have lost some or all of their hearing. These specially trained dogs are taught to make physical contact with their owners in response to a variety of daily sounds. "When the phone rings, someone knocks on the door, or an alarm sounds, the dog finds the owner, jumps up, and starts pawing her legs to get her attention," says Michael Sapp, chief operating officer of PAWS with a Cause in Wayland, Michigan. "Then the dog either takes the owner to the source of the sound or, in the case of a fire alarm, leads her out of the house."

Most service dogs are large breeds such as shepherds or retrievers, but hearing dogs tend to be small breeds, Sapp says. "If the phone rings, you don't want a 90-pound rottweiler jumping up on you to let you know."

with one type of behavior, he'll naturally try other things that please you more.

Trainers used to recommend raising a knee to discourage persistent jumpers. The idea was to bump their chests, reducing the momentum and giving them an uncomfortable jolt. The problem with this technique is that a knee raised too forcefully can hurt a dog. Most experts now believe that it's better to use the force of your authority—and your voice—than to get physical.

Give praise and more praise. "Dogs don't really know what to do until you show them by praising them when they behave in a way that you like," says Cathy Jobe, founder of Waterloo Farms, a dog-training facility in Celina, Texas. You don't want to give your dog attention or affection while he's jumping up. You do want to shower him with praise when he greets you calmly or sits when you tell him to. "Dogs want to be good," she explains. "But the only way they know when they are being good is when you praise them."

Come down to his level. Your dog craves face-to-face interaction. Dogs try to close the height gap in the only way they can—by jumping up. "Dogs also can find our height a bit intimidating," says Ira B. Perelle, Ph.D., a certified applied animal behaviorist and chairperson of the development committee for the Animal Behavior Society in Bloomington, Indiana. "It's a real pleasure for our pets when we sit down and interact closely with them," he says. "I try to crouch or sit as much as possible when I'm among four-legged animals."

Show by example. We practically invite jumping when we make a huge production about coming home. "Dogs pick up on the excitement levels of those around them," says Stephen Zawistowski, Ph.D., a certified applied animal behaviorist and a senior vice president of animal services and science advisor for the American Society for the Prevention of Cruelty to Animals in New York City. "If you come in the door making a commotion, waving your arms, and being very loud, it's understandable that your dog will respond by jumping up."

Help your dog stay calm by being calm yourself. When you come home, give your dog a warm but sedate hello. Then go about your business for a while. Only when you've settled in and the usual homecoming energy is lower should you give your dog your full attention.

Leash Pulling

Dogs have very strong independent streaks. As much as they love you, they certainly have no natural interest in being bound to your side by a strip of leather. This is why a puppy's first reaction is to pull away when a leash is clipped on his collar.

"If you haven't taken the time to train your dog not to pull on a leash, you can't blame him for jerking you around," says John Fioramonti, D.V.M., a veterinarian in Towson, Maryland. Training isn't the whole story, however.

Sometimes pulling occurs when dogs are out on a walk and see other dogs. They're not sure whether or not these strangers are friendly. So they put on quite a display to make sure the dogs know that you're being protected, says Joanne Hibbs, D.V.M., a veterinarian in Knoxville, Tennessee.

Pulling on the leash in this situation isn't likely to calm them down, Dr. Hibbs adds. In fact, your dog may interpret tension on the leash as meaning "I'm scared." Being a good dog, he'll throw herself against the leash even harder in an attempt to confront the threat head-on.

Other times, dogs get so excited about their walks that they pull like crazy in order to see and sniff all the exciting stuff out there. This happens even with well-behaved dogs, Dr. Fioramonti adds. They're not deliberately ignoring your tugs and commands. They're just so caught up in the moment that they've forgotten you're attached to the other end of the leash.

Dogs that pull only when they're over-the-top excited are pretty easy to rein in, says Ken Nagler, a trainer in Beltsville, Maryland. But just pulling on the leash won't help because dogs will pull back without even thinking about it, he adds. If, however, you vary your pace when you're out on walks by suddenly speeding up, slowing down, or making a tight turn, your dog will keep watching you just to see what's going to happen next.

Think of the leash as a telephone wire that carries messages back and forth. By paying attention to your own signals and also reading your dog's, you can make the leash act more as a communications device than as a restraint. Here's what experts recommend.

The Solutions

Check the distance. Unless you're training your dog for the show ring, it probably doesn't matter if he walks in perfect heeling position. Every dog, however, tends to walk a certain distance away from his owner. You can tell your dog's mind is wandering when he's walking farther ahead or farther behind than usual. This is the time to change direction, call his name, or pat your leg, says Nagler. As long as your dog is interacting with and focusing on you, he won't be looking for distractions.

Reward a loose leash. Dogs don't do anything for free. At the very least, they expect to be rewarded with approval; food is even better. So put a few biscuits in your

Different Dogs, Different Collars

Dogs that heel perfectly all the time don't need anything more than flat leather or nylon buckle-up collars. Those that are persistent pullers, however, may need training collars. Here are the options.

Choke collars. These act like fast-release nooses. When you give a sharp tug, the collar quickly tightens and gets a dog's attention. The pressure instantly releases when you relax your hold on the leash. Choke collars tell dogs, "Pay attention *now*."

Pinch collars. These act like choke collars, but they're equipped with flat-tipped prongs that normally lie flat so dogs don't feel them. When you pull on the leash, however, the prongs come together and pinch and poke the skin around the neck. The pinch is hard to ignore, and even headstrong dogs quit pulling in order to avoid it.

Head halters. There are several brands, such as the Gentle Leader. Unlike collars, which encircle the neck, head halters have straps that slip over the muzzle and across the back of the neck, then fasten with a ring under the chin. Since the pressure is distributed over the entire head, it's much easier to guide your dog. In addition, the halters put pressure on the back of the neck and on the muzzle—the same spots that mother dogs grab when their puppies misbehave.

You can get these halters from veterinarians, trainers, and behaviorists. They need to be professionally fitted, and you'll get instructions on how to use them properly.

pocket when you go for walks. As long as your dog is walking nicely and the leash is slack, stop now and then and give him something to eat, Nagler suggests. He won't think about it, but unconsciously he'll start to associate his behavior and your respective body positions with nice treats. After a while, he'll automatically walk with less pulling.

Pull fast, not slow. The message you send while pulling on the leash depends on how you pull it. To prevent a tug-of-war with the leash, it's better to give a sharp, fast pull, then immediately let the leash go slack. "Pulling slowly sometimes makes dogs gag, which sounds terrible, but they couldn't care less," Nagler says. "They just ignore it and pull harder." A sharp tug, by contrast, instantly gets their attention and lets them know there's something you want, he explains.

Consider the breed. Samoyeds, huskies, and malamutes were bred to be sled dogs. Rottweilers and giant schnauzers are the descendants of carting dogs. And terriers just enjoy challenges; pulling things gives them a real kick. You can't change dogs' natures, but you can give them a chance to get the pulling urge out of their systems, Nagler says.

You can buy dog carts and harnesses from some specialty catalogs, such as Dog Works in Stewartstown, Pennsylvania. Some people even hook their canine Clydesdales to child-size push scooters and let them pull them up the sidewalk. Once they've burned off some of that energy and satisfied their instincts, they'll be much less likely to pull the leash, Nagler says.

Start early. "I like to clip a leash on a puppy almost as soon as I bring him home," says Nagler. You don't even have to hold the leash at first. Just let it drag as your puppy gets used to it.

Encourage him to come to you. Puppies don't always do what people want, and coming when they're called isn't necessarily as interesting as going the other way. When you're ready to start leash training your puppy, and he's dragging the leash behind him, crouch down low, then pick up the leash as you call his name. The tug will get his attention, and your low position and pleasant tone will invite him to play, says Dr. Hibbs.

Your pup should run toward you, tail wagging. If he balks, resist the urge to reel him in like a fish. That will just get him used to feeling a tight leash, Dr. Hibbs says.

People first. "If you always go through the door or into the car before your puppy, you'll set the stage for obedience on the leash," says Nagler. Puppies that run ahead of people when they're off-leash are going to do the same thing when they're on one, he explains.

Licking

For pets, the tongue is more than an eating utensil. It's a handy tool for grooming, cleaning wounds, and expressing affection and social ties. They spend so much time licking, in fact, that any decrease in tongue action usually means that they're sick, says Benjamin Hart, D.V.M., Ph.D., professor of physiology and behavior at the University of California, Davis, School of Veterinary Medicine and author of *The Perfect Puppy: How to Choose Your Dog by Its Behavior*. Researchers believe that some of the same changes in the body that accompany a fever, for example, may temporarily reduce the licking instinct.

Cats spend enormous amounts of time licking their fur as part of their grooming rituals. Dogs are renowned for how much they lick others. People often suspect that salty skin is what draws their dogs closer, but licking isn't about taste, says Dr. Hart. They do it because they like us. Dogs also use their tongues to communicate a variety of messages, such as that they're hungry.

Veterinarians aren't sure why some dogs and cats get almost compulsive about licking. They'll groom themselves so often that their fur is perpetually damp. Or they'll lick so long and vigorously that they develop painful, slow-to-heal sores called lick granulomas, says Myrna Milani, D.V.M., a veterinarian in Charlestown, New Hampshire, and author of *DogSmart* and *CatSmart*.

Stress almost certainly plays a role in over-the-top licking, says Dr. Hart. Pets respond to stress by licking their fur, just as people sometimes respond to stress by biting their nails. Even when the original source of stress is long gone, they may keep licking just because it has become a habit. There's also a theory that pets have an internal grooming clock. It's possible that this mechanism may become overactive, stimulating cats and dogs to lick more than they usually would.

Compulsive licking is always a problem, not only because it can damage the skin but also because it's a sign that something in their lives is out of balance, says Dr. Hart. Veterinarians usually recommend the following four-step program to stop excessive licking.

The Solutions

Try to figure out what's setting them off. Dogs and cats don't adjust to change very well, and licking is often their response to something new or different. Getting a new pet may trigger licking in the resident pet, says Dr. Hart. So will making an outdoor cat become an indoor cat. Even changes in your routine, such as spending more time away from home, can result in nervous licking. Helping pets adjust to change, which often involves nothing more than time, patience, and a little extra attention, may be enough to stop the problem.

Keep them occupied. "Some people find that it helps to add some structure to the animal's environment," says Dr.

Hart. This can be as simple as scheduling exercise once or twice a day. Better yet, do a little training or teach your pets some tricks. Interacting with people and the mental stimulation of learning new things is usually enough to take their minds off their coats.

Break the habit by redirecting their attention. Even when dogs and cats are feeling calm and happy, they'll sometimes continue licking because at some time in the past they got accustomed to calming themselves with this behavior. Habits are hard to break, and pets often need some help redirecting their attention to other, less harmful activities, says Kimberly Barry, Ph.D., a certified applied

Not As Bad As It Seems

People cringe when they think of all the things—dirt, mucky water, and other bits of nastiness—that dogs and cats lick from their coats every day. While a tongueful of dirt isn't very hygienic, nature made sure that dogs and cats are up to the task. Their saliva and digestive systems can handle just about anything they lick up. "They have pretty powerful systems that can get rid of nasty things we might think twice about consuming," says Benjamin Hart, D.V.M., Ph.D., professor of physiology and behavior at the University of California, Davis, School of Veterinary Medicine and author of *The Perfect Puppy: How to Choose Your Dog by Its Behavior*.

Parasites, bacteria, and fungi don't have much chance of surviving, he explains. And because dogs and cats have saliva that acts as a mild disinfectant, their habit of licking their wounds can help prevent infection-causing germs from multiplying.

animal behaviorist in Austin, Texas. As soon as you notice your pet licking, distract her by making a noise, then give her a toy or play with her for a while, she advises. The fewer opportunities she has to lick herself, the easier it will be for her to give up the habit.

Ask about drug therapy. It isn't always needed, but drug therapy can be very helpful for pets that are constantly licking. Drugs help adjust the balance of chemicals in the brain, which can stop repetitive behavior, says Dr. Milani. Some pets will need to stay on medications, but most of the time they're only needed for a month or two and are used to supplement behavior therapy, she explains.

Skin Chewing

Dogs and cats spend a lot of time grooming—everything from licking their bellies to nibbling their toes. But when their skin is itchy or irritated, they won't leave it alone. They act as though their paws, tails, or flanks are corn on the cob, chewing so vigorously and for so long that they wear away the fur or even damage the skin.

Chewing usually begins when pets are sensitive to something in the environment, like pollen, fleas, or chemicals in their food, says Steven A. Melman, V.M.D., a veterinarian with practices in Potomac, Maryland, and Palm Springs, California, and author of *Skin Diseases of Dogs and Cats*. Even when the original problem is gone, dogs and cats may keep chewing out of habit, especially when they are stressed or bored.

Skin problems can be complicated to treat, so it is a good idea to talk to your vet when problems begin. In the meantime, here are a few natural, drug-free ways to take a bite out of chewing.

The Solutions

Rinse away problems. Rinsing pets with cool water once a day will wash away dust, pollen, and other substances that may cause itching and skin chewing, says Dr. Melman. You can gently spray dogs with a garden hose or a spray nozzle in the bathtub. It is especially helpful to wash their feet after they have been outside. Cats aren't thrilled about water in any form, but they particularly hate being sprayed. So you may have to bathe them with water instead, he says.

Use a natural shampoo. When a plain water rinse doesn't stop the itch, you may want to try a soothing all-natural shampoo made with oatmeal, says Carolyn Blakey, D.V.M., a holistic veterinarian in private practice in Richmond, Indiana. Make sure that the shampoo doesn't contain dyes, fragrances, or animal proteins, which can trigger

Call the Vet

Most dogs and cats have occasional itchy spells. Itching that doesn't go away fairly quickly should always be checked out by a veterinarian, says Steven A. Melman, V.M.D., a veterinarian with practices in Potomac, Maryland, and Palm Springs, California, and author of *Skin Diseases of Dogs and Cats*. There are a number of serious conditions, from hard-to-treat emotional problems to internal illnesses, that can cause constant chewing. Some dogs and cats will go as far as to chew their skin raw, he adds.

"If you find yourself using a home treatment like a cool-water bath more often than once a day for 3 or 4 days, you have to see your vet," says Dr. Melman.

allergic reactions, Dr. Melman adds. And rinse out the soap thoroughly when you are done. Even small amounts of residual suds will cause itching when they dry.

Soothe the emotions. It is very common for dogs and cats to chew their skin during times of stress, says Dr. Blakey. To help them feel more tranquil, she recommends giving 4 drops of the flower essence crab apple. You can put the drops directly in their mouths or into their water bowls once a day.

Apply a soothing ointment. Hypericum, the active ingredient in St. John's wort, may help reduce itching that causes skin chewing, says Susan G. Wynn, D.V.M., a veterinarian in Atlanta and coeditor of *Complementary and Alternative Veterinary Medicine*. Apply it to your pet's skin twice a day, she says. The ointment is available in health food stores.

Counter the itch with a Chinese cure. Specialists in traditional Chinese medicine sometimes recommend a product called Armadillo Counter-Poison Pill. "It combines several herbs, and it works as well as antihistamines to soothe itchy skin," says Michelle Tilghman, D.V.M., a holistic veterinarian in private practice in Stone Mountain, Georgia. She recommends giving pets under 15 pounds one tablet twice a day. Pets 15 to 50 pounds can take two tablets twice a day, and larger pets can take three tablets twice a day.

Calm the skin with an herbal blend. A product called Hokamix, available from veterinarians and mail-order catalogs, contains a variety of herbs that reduce skin inflammation and help the body fight allergies that can cause chewing, says Nancy Scanlan, D.V.M., a holistic veterinarian in private practice in Sherman Oaks, California. Mix the Hokamix with their food, following the directions that come in the box. Most pets like the taste, so you won't have to work to disguise it, she adds.

Use a homeopathic combo. Health food and pet supply stores stock a variety of homeopathic remedies for stop-

Cater to Your Cat

Cats hate being sprayed with water even more than they hate baths, so the best way to rinse pollen and other allergens off your cat's coat is to slowly lower her (one hand supporting her bottom, the other beneath the chest) into a sink half filled with water. Restrain her firmly by the back of the neck and ladle water over her with a cup. Putting a small towel in the bottom of the sink will give her traction so that she is less likely to slip.

ping itch-related chewing, such as HomeoPet Hot Spot Dermatitis or HomeoPet Skin and Seborrhea. "They are typically low-potency pills that contain a combination of remedies, and at least one of the ingredients is likely to help," says Dr. Blakey. Dogs can take 10 drops and cats can have 3 drops, both three times a day. Call your vet if your pet keeps chewing, she says.

Feed them naturally. The artificial dyes and flavorings in many commercial pet foods often cause itchy skin, says Dr. Blakey. Most holistic veterinarians recommend giving pets all-natural diets—either diets made from scratch or commercial foods such as Wysong or Innova.

Soothe the skin with fish-oil supplements. Fish oil contains omega-3 fatty acids, which help relieve irritation that can lead to skin chewing, says Dr. Wynn. Give cats and dogs weighing under 20 pounds 500 milligrams a day, she says. Pets 20 to 50 pounds can take 1,000 to 2,000 milligrams. Dogs 51 to 80 pounds can take 3,000 milligrams, and larger dogs can have 4,000 milligrams. Oils made from the whole fish, like salmon oil, are a good choice because they contain more omega-3 fatty acids than those made from just a part of the fish, like cod-liver oil.

Spraying and Marking

Like urban graffiti, a cat's urine spray is meant to grab attention. It helps attract mates and drive away male competition, says Nicholas Dodman, B.V.M.S. (bachelor of veterinary medicine and surgery, a British equivalent of D.V.M.), professor of behavioral pharmacology and director of the behavior clinic at Tufts University School of Veterinary Medicine in North Grafton, Massachusetts. Spraying is most common in males, although females sometimes do it, too. Some cats also spray to boost their confidence when they are feeling insecure and anxious.

Dogs do things differently. They have a way of turning even short walks into time-consuming marathons, especially when they insist on pausing at every tree, bush, and light pole to empty their bladders a teaspoonful at a time.

"When a dog lifts his leg against a tree, he's not just relieving himself," says Liz Palika, a trainer in Oceanside, California. "He's also marking the tree with his scent, leaving his calling card for every dog that passes by after him."

No one would complain too much if cats and dogs did their marking outside. But sometimes they bring this habit indoors or right around the house and begin marking decks, porches, doors, and garage doors. Cat urine is especially pungent, and the stench—produced by an odorific soup of chemical compounds, including uric acid and pheromones—can linger for weeks.

Here are some natural ways to get control of the situation.

The Solutions

Calm cats with good scents. A cat's urine is filled with pheromones, natural chemicals that convey signals of anxiety, anger, or aggression. The pheromones in the facial glands, by contrast, convey messages of peace and contentment. Because cats won't spray in "happy" places, you can often control spraying by overwriting the urine marks with a product called Feliway, which contains chemicals similar to those in the facial glands, says Alison Clarke, V.M.D., a retired veterinarian in Leonardtown, Maryland. After washing the urine marks, she recommends spraying them with the pheromones twice a day for about a month, then once or twice a week thereafter. Feliway is available from veterinarians.

Soothe anxiety. Since spraying cats are often anxious cats, flower essences can help make them calmer and more secure, says Arthur Young, D.V.M., a holistic veterinarian in private practice in Stuart, Florida. He recommends putting a drop of the essence Bach Rescue Remedy on the skin on the inner part of each earflap four times a day. In addition, you may want to mix flower essences in your cat's drinking water. Put 2 drops each of Bach Rescue Remedy, chestnut bud, vervain, and vine in his water each day, Dr. Young advises.

Battle it with boxes. Anxiety sometimes begins at the litter box, especially if you live in a multiple-cat household. Giving each cat his own box will help keep them all content, says Dr. Clarke. "You absolutely need at least one litter pan per cat. Often, anything less causes cats to spray."

It is also helpful to put the litter boxes in different parts of the house rather than all lined up in a row. This gives each cat privacy and reduces the possibility of squabbles over squatting rights.

Clean naturally. Cats dislike chemical smells, and using household cleaners on the litter box will often make spraying worse. Ammonia-based cleaners are especially offensive because, to cats, they smell like the urine of another cat. Your pet may start spraying in order to warn off the phantom intruder. "I've never found anything better than plain soap and water for basic cleaning," says Dr. Clarke.

Neutralize the smell. Often cats that get in the habit of spraying return to the same spots for a bit of urine renewal. Scrubbing will remove most of the smell, but invariably a few molecules will be left behind. Dr. Clarke recommends soaking the area with an odor neutralizer, such as Nature's Miracle. Odor neutralizers contain natural enzymes or bacteria that break down the chemicals in the urine.

Treat your cat kindly. Cats don't spray out of spite but merely to obey powerful physical or emotional needs, says Gary Landsberg, D.V.M., a veterinary behaviorist in private practice in Thornhill, Ontario. It doesn't help to punish cats by yelling or stamping your feet. In fact, getting angry will make your cat even more insecure—and more likely to spray. The best approach is to give him all the love and attention you can and reward him with a treat or a few strokes whenever he uses his box instead of the wall, he advises.

Call the Vet

There are a number of physical problems, such as diabetes or urinary tract infections, that can cause cats to spray. It is always worth taking him to the vet for a checkup before you try to treat the problem at home, says Gary Landsberg, D.V.M., a veterinary behaviorist in private practice in Thornhill, Ontario.

Don't waste time when your pet starts spraying, Dr. Landsberg adds. Some cats, once they get in the habit, have a hard time giving it up. "Take that first spray very seriously," he says. "Whisk him right off to the vet to see if there is a physical problem and to nip the habit in the bud."

Keep them moving. It's normal for dogs to mark trees and bushes on their walks. For dogs with somewhat dominant personalities, however, the freedom to mark at will can make them more dominant and harder to handle. "Being allowed to mark the entire neighborhood as his home turf can make a dog even more aggressive," says Larry Lachman, Ph.D., an animal-behavior consultant based in Carmel, California, and author of *Dogs on the Couch* and *Cats on the Counter*. He recommends picking one or two spots along your usual route where you always let your dog stop. The rest of the time, keep him moving, he says.

Tell them what you think. Pets are eager to please their people, which means they'll often quit doing things they know make you unhappy. It doesn't do any good to punish them after they've made a mess, says Bonnie Beaver, D.V.M., a board-certified veterinary behaviorist, certified applied animal behaviorist, professor of animal behavior at Texas A&M University College of Veterinary Medicine in College Station, and author of *Feline Behavior: A Guide for Veterinarians*. Dogs and cats have short memories and probably won't know what you're mad about.

"The best way to help pets understand that you don't like their behavior is to catch them in the act and firmly tell them no," says Wayne Hunthausen, D.V.M., a veterinary behaviorist in Westwood, Kansas, and coauthor of *Handbook of Behaviour Problems of the Dog and Cat*. If that doesn't make your pet stop, clap your hands or slap your palm against a table. As soon as he looks at you, put him to work. Tell him to lie down or sit for a while. For cats, hold them for a minute. You don't want to praise or reward them, but it's important not to let them finish what they started, he says. Dogs and cats are creatures of habit, and the longer you can keep them from marking, the less likely they'll be to continue doing it.

Incidentally, don't let your cat see you when you're making a sharp sound. "Cats don't recover from verbal discipline as quickly as dogs," Dr. Hunthausen says. You don't want your cat to blame you for scaring him.

Take away the opportunity. Since cats often spray in the same place, you can discourage them by rearranging the room so that the area is out of reach—behind a piece of furniture, for example. Better yet, Palika recommends putting your cat's food and water bowls near where he's spraying. Cats are very reluctant to make messes in places they associate with food and good times.

"If your dog is prone to marking indoors, don't allow him free run of the house when you're not around to watch him," suggests Palika. "Confine him to a kennel or crate when you're gone, and keep him in the same room with you at other times." Dogs that aren't used to crates don't always take to them easily, she adds, so talk to your veterinarian before shutting your dog in for the first time.

Ask about neutering. Pets that are spayed or neutered—veterinarians usually recommend doing it when they're less than 6 months old—are much less likely to spray or mark than their intact counterparts, says Dr. Hunthausen. Neutering is more effective in cats than in dogs. About 50 percent of male dogs will continue to mark after neutering, says Dr. Hunthausen. Only about 10 percent of male cats, however, will continue to mark and spray after neutering.

Wool Sucking

Veterinarians aren't sure why, but some cats become almost obsessed with sucking and chewing on fabrics, a condition known as wool sucking. Some cats may do it because they were abandoned or left the nest too early, and sucking on fabric reminds them of the comfort of nursing. Emotional stress or nutritional deficiencies may play a role. And since cats look entirely blissful while chewing on wool (or any other fabric), it may be nothing more than an act of pure pleasure.

Wool sucking is actually more of a people problem than a pet problem since the main threat is to your belongings. But sucking sometimes turns to chewing, and chewing can turn to swallowing—and that is when the behavior starts getting dangerous for the animal. Veterinarians sometimes treat wool sucking with medications such as fluoxetine (Prozac), which can help curtail many types of compulsive behavior. Before turning to powerful drugs, however, you may want to try a few simpler and safer approaches.

The Solutions

Satisfy the craving. Since cats that chew wool are thought to crave crunch, you may be able to break the habit by giving them a crunchy substitute such as lettuce, says John C. Wright, Ph.D., a certified applied animal behaviorist; professor of psychology at Mercer University in Macon, Georgia; and author of *The Dog Who Would Be King* and *Is Your Cat Crazy?* Carrots or dry kibble may also satisfy their need for an *al dente* diet.

Give them a garden of their own. Another way to keep cats out of the closets is to put up a window box filled with catnip or grass. Cats love natural greenery, and the extra dietary fiber may decrease the urge to chew wool. "Cats tend to go through kitty gardens like lawn mowers," says Vint Virga, D.V.M., a veterinarian at the behavior clinic at Cornell University College of Veterinary Medicine in Ithaca, New York. You can buy window gardens made especially for cats in pet supply stores and some garden stores.

Keep them busy. People often forget that cats are high-octane animals that evolved as hunters, jumpers, and climbers. They need a lot of exercise, and if they don't get it, they look for other ways to blow off steam, such as gnawing their way through the linens, says Kimberly Barry, Ph.D., a certified applied animal behaviorist in Austin, Texas.

Most cats don't go for walks the way dogs do, but they love to sprint—after a dragged piece of string, for example, or the light from a laser pointer. (Laser light is intense, so keep it away from their eyes.) And nearly every cat loves batting balled-up pieces of paper. You can make the crumpled paper even more exciting by hiding some food inside, says Dr. Barry.

Make life predictable. Humans adapt quickly to change, but cats don't, says Linda Goodloe, Ph.D., a certified applied animal behaviorist in New York City. Even small changes in routines, like moving the litter box to another room, can make cats anxious, and anxious cats sometimes start chewing.

You can try to minimize the types of disruptions that make them upset. Two things that cats care most about are regular meals and a clean litter box, Dr. Goodloe says. Keeping these two things predictable will help them weather most other changes that come their way.

Distract them with something better. You can train cats to leave your belongings alone as long as you distract them right away, says Dr. Goodloe. Whenever you see your cat chewing, clap your hands or make some other noise to get his attention. Then flick a ball or a length of string across his peripheral vision—an area cats closely watch because that's where mice and other prey appear. Once he starts playing, give him a reward—either a food treat or simply more play. He'll learn that he has more fun playing with you than chewing in private, she explains.

Change the taste. Pet supply stores sell products such as Grannick's Bitter Apple, which you can spray on areas your cat is chewing. The repellents are fabric safe and have tastes cats dislike. Or you could sprinkle black pepper on your cat's object of choice. (As an alternative, dissolve black pepper in hot water, let it cool, then spray it in places where you don't want him to go.) You can't coat your entire house, but most cats have a few favorite items that they return to again and again. Treating these items may convince your cat that *all* fabrics now have that yucky taste.

Another taste technique is to pour rubbing alcohol or Bitter Apple, along with a splash of your usual cologne, on a piece of clothing or linen that your cat has already destroyed. Then lightly scent other articles of clothing with the cologne alone. The idea is for your cat to chew on his usual item and get a bad taste along with a noseful of cologne. He may connect the two and assume that anything that smells like cologne is not for him, says Dr. Wright.

Upgrade his diet. Some cats may start sucking or chewing material because their diets aren't providing all the nutrients they need. "They could have a need for trace minerals," says Michael W. Lemmon, D.V.M., a holistic veterinarian in Renton, Washington, and past president of the American Holistic Veterinary Medical Association.

He recommends changing your cat's diet, giving him 75 percent organic raw meat and 25 percent raw vegetables, such as carrots. In addition, you should mix in his food ¼ to ½ teaspoon of powdered sea vegetables, such as kelp or dulse, which are rich in trace minerals. Try the diet for about a month. If your cat becomes less materially inclined, he probably just needs a higher-quality food, he says.

Give him more fiber. Cats need dietary fiber just as much as people do, and they may start gnawing material to replace fiber that is missing in their diets, says Dr. Lemmon. He recommends mixing a teaspoon of oat bran, wheat bran, or flaxseed in your cat's food every day.

Calm his nerves with homeopathy. There are a number of homeopathic remedies that can help ease the anxiety that can lead to wool sucking. For example, Silica 6X, given twice a day for 7 days, can help stop wool sucking in cats that are also nervous or shy, says Robin Cannizzaro, D.V.M., a holistic veterinarian in private practice in St. Petersburg, Florida. The usual dose is 2 or 3 drops of liquid Silica or four to five pellets. If your cat isn't getting better within a week, call a holistic veterinarian for advice, she recommends.

Relieve his anxiety. Since cats may turn to wool during times of tension, give your cat calming herbs, such as St. John's wort (*Hypericum perforatum*) or kava kava (*Piper methysticum*), says Dr. Cannizzaro. "You can use a product that combines the two herbs, or you can give them separately." St. John's wort may cause side effects in some pets, however, so talk to your vet before using it at home. If it is going to work, you should see results in about 2 weeks, she adds.

Try healing essences. Flower remedies can be very helpful for cats that are sucking wool if they are nervous or upset, says Christina Chambreau, D.V.M., a holistic veterinarian in Sparks, Maryland, and education chairperson for the Academy of Veterinary Homeopathy. "A cat that is tense and anxious, for example, might need vervain," she says. "One that is fearful and timid might need aspen and mimulus. A cat that starts wool sucking after another animal is added to the household may need holly for jealousy." You may want to try chestnut bud as well since it is a common remedy for stopping repetitious behavior.

To prepare the remedies, put 2 drops of an essence in a 1-ounce dropper bottle filled with pure water. Shake it 10 to 20 times and give your cat one dropperful three or four times a day. You can put the drops in his mouth or in his drinking water. "You should notice some improvement within 2 weeks," says Dr. Chambreau. "It is a good idea to continue giving it for a month or two, then resume it later if the behavior starts to recur."

Resources

First-Aid: When Every Minute Counts

Dogs and cats just don't think about danger. That's why our knowing first-aid is so important.

"Knowing how to take quick, calm action can literally spell the difference between life and death," says Joseph Trueba, D.V.M., a veterinarian in Tucson, Arizona, who specializes in emergency care. You don't have to be a trained paramedic, but you do have to be prepared—emotionally and mentally—to do *something*. Even if your vet is only minutes away, knowing what to do in the moments right after an injury occurs can make all the difference.

Having a well-stocked first-aid kit is critical, says Dr. Trueba. You'll find everything you need in "Making a First-Aid Kit" on page 255. You also have to be prepared to stop bleeding, move your pet safely, or even do CPR. The following pages cover some of the most common emergencies. If you there are any instructions you don't understand, have your vet demonstrate proper technique—before you need it.

Muzzling an Injured Pet

"Once injured, any pet can become a ferocious biter or scratcher," warns Dr. Trueba. "Always protect yourself first or you won't be able to help your pet."

Veterinarians recommend muzzling dogs and cats before performing first-aid. You can buy a ready-made muzzle at pet supply stores and keep it in your first-aid kit. Or you can make one on the spot by using a long strip of gauze or even your pet's leash. Here's how to use gauze.

To muzzle a dog. Because of their longer snouts, dogs are a bit easier to muzzle than cats.

1. Starting with a piece of gauze about 24 inches long, make a loop in the middle, then cross the ends over each other and then run the ends through the loop, as if you're beginning to tie a bow on a pair of shoes.
2. Slide the loop over your dog's snout with the ends of the gauze on top. Pull it taut about halfway up his nose.
3. Carry the ends under the chin and make a square knot.
4. Bring the ends behind his ears and tie a bow for quick release.

To muzzle a cat. "While a muzzle generally provides sufficient restraint for a dog, you may have to further subdue your cat to avoid getting scratched," says Joan E. Antle, D.V.M., a veterinarian in private practice in Cleveland.

1. Wrap your cat in a towel, leaving room for her to breathe. Using a strip of gauze about 20 inches long, make a loop in the middle, then cross the ends over each other and then through the loop, as if you're beginning to tie a bow on a pair of shoes.
2. Place the loop around your cat's nose as far back as possible, leaving the ends under the chin.
3. Tighten the loop and pull the ends behind her ears. Tie the ends firmly in a square knot at the nape of the neck.

4. Bring one end of the strip down and loop it under the nose loop. Carry it back once again to the nape of the neck and tie the ends in a bow for quick release.

Moving an Injured Pet

If your dog or cat is seriously injured—having been hit by a car, for example—you are going to have to move her either to the side of the road or into the backseat of your car for the ride to the vet. Moving a pet with neck, back, or spinal cord injuries, however, can be as dangerous to your pet as the accident itself. It's essential to do it right.

To move your pet quickly, grasp her by the nape of the neck with one hand and by the skin of the hips with the other and drag her out of harm's way, advises Dr. Antle. You don't want to lift her off the ground because that can put dangerous pressure on the injured areas.

Time permitting, a pet with serious injuries should be immobilized before moving, says Dr. Antle. By moving her as one "unit," without allowing the spine or legs to move, you can help prevent further damage while you are getting your pet to the vet. It's easy to immobilize cats and small dogs—they can be lifted smoothly into a box or pet carrier. For large dogs, however, you are going to need a whole-body splint. Here are two approaches.

- Being careful not to bend the spine, neck, or legs, drag your pet onto a firm surface like a piece of plywood with a sheet spread beneath it. Cover her with the sheet and tie her down by knotting the ends of the sheet around the board.
- If you don't have a board handy, you can fashion a makeshift stretcher by taking a blanket or sheet and folding it in half. Drag your pet onto the blanket, then roll up the sides to take up the slack and form handles.

Stopping Bleeding

Most bleeding is caused by something minor—a piece of glass in a paw, for instance. "A little blood can look like a lot because it spreads quickly," says Dr. Antle. You can stop most bleeding by pressing on the area with a piece of gauze. (If blood soaks through the gauze, add some more. Don't remove the gauze because it may disturb clots that are trying to form.) Then it's just a matter of cleaning up the mess.

Bleeding that is unusually heavy or that doesn't stop within a few minutes needs more serious attention. Vets recommend keeping pressure on the wound by taping on a piece of gauze, for example, while also using your three middle fingers to push down on one of your pet's pressure points. These points are the areas between the wound and the heart where a little finger pressure will partially collapse an artery, causing bleeding to slow. Here are where the major pressure points exist:

- where the lower jaw meets the ear
- in the soft groove next to your pet's windpipe
- under the armpit
- in the middle of the groin, where the thigh meets the body
- under the base of the tail.

If you're unsure of the location of these pressure points, have your vet show you exactly where they are.

Regardless of the pressure point you use, be sure to relax the pressure for 1 or 2 seconds every 10 seconds. This permits some blood to get through, which will keep surrounding tissues healthy, Dr. Antle says. Wounds that are bleeding this heavily always require professional care, she adds, so get your pet to the vet as soon as possible.

Using a Tourniquet Safely

For years, first-aid manuals recommended applying a tourniquet to stop bleeding. Today most vets don't like them. Unless they are used properly, they can make things worse by restricting bloodflow to healthy tissues around the wound.

When you can't stop bleeding any other way, however, a tourniquet could save your pet's life. "Always use it as a last resort and only on a leg or tail," says Craig N. Carter, D.V.M., Ph.D., head of epidemiology at the Texas Veterinary Medical Diagnostic Laboratory at Texas A&M University in College Station. As soon as the tourniquet is in place, get your pet to the vet immediately.

1. Wrap a strip of cloth twice around the leg or tail between the bleeding and the heart, but don't knot it.
2. Place a stick, pencil, or any other hard, straight object on top of the second layer of cloth and tie it in place with the two loose ends.
3. Twist the stick to tighten the tourniquet. It should be just tight enough to stop the bleeding. *Be sure to loosen the tourniquet for 1 to 2 seconds every 10 seconds.* This will allow blood to flow and nourish healthy tissues while still keeping the bleeding under control.

Administering CPR

If your dog or cat has been in an accident, the heart and lungs may quit working. Once this happens, you have only 3 to 5 minutes to restore the flow of oxygen to the brain to prevent permanent damage.

The best way to save your pet is with cardiopulmonary resuscitation, or CPR. "It's always worth trying CPR on your pet if he has stopped breathing and there is no immediate medical assistance," says Craig N. Carter, D.V.M., Ph.D., head of epidemiology at the Texas Veterinary Medical Diagnostic Laboratory at Texas A&M University in College Station. Even if you are en route to the vet, you (or a car passenger) should be prepared to do CPR until you get there.

Here's how to do it right.

1. **Open the airway.** Using your index and middle finger, swipe any material out of your pet's mouth, being careful in case she bites. In some cases, this may be enough to clear a blocked airway and start her breathing again. If she still can't breathe, check to be sure that her neck isn't crimped. She should be lying on her side, with her head in line with the neck. Pull the tongue forward to see if breathing resumes.

2. **Help her breathe.** If your pet doesn't start breathing on her own, hold her mouth shut and place your mouth over the nostrils. Blow into the nose two times, using just enough force to make the chest rise. (Blowing too hard can overinflate the lungs of small pets.) If the chest doesn't rise, reposition the neck and try again. If you can't get the chest to rise, you may need to do the Heimlich maneuver. (For more information, see "Choking" on page 253.)

3. **Circulate blood.** Lay your pet on her right side. Place the heel of one hand over the ribs on the pet's left side. Your hand should be roughly over the heart. Place your other hand over the first, and, using both hands, press down with enough force to compress the chest. For small dogs and cats, compress the chest ½ inch. For medium dogs, the chest should compress 1 inch; and for large dogs, it should go down 1½ inches. Vets recommend compressing the chest 15 times. Then breathe into the nose twice and start pressing on the chest again. Continue this until your pet starts breathing on her own again or until you can get her to the vet.

Bites

"Bites are often deep, and they are loaded with bacteria that can start an infection quickly," Dr. Antle says. "It's best to take your pet to the vet, who can clean the wound properly." Washing bite wounds at home often drives dirt and bacteria in deeper, making the injury worse.

One of the hidden dangers of bite wounds is simply their small size; they are not always easy to see. This means an infection may be quietly forming, getting worse every day. If you see an area that is red, swollen, or warm to the touch, call your vet right away. "Infected wounds need emergency veterinary care," says Dr. Antle. This is especially true if your pet has been spending time outdoors. Rabies isn't very common in dogs and cats, but it is common in skunks, raccoons, foxes, bats, and other wild animals. Your pet may need fast treatment.

Burns

Thankfully, most burns aren't serious and can be treated at home the same way you would treat your own—by applying an ice cube or a cold pack or by flooding the area with cold water. "Applying cold stops a burn from penetrating into deeper tissues," explains Paul M. Gigliotti, D.V.M., a veterinarian in private practice in Mayfield Village, Ohio. "Apply the cold treatment for a full 20 minutes after the burn," he says.

If the area is red and swollen, however, follow the cold treatment by applying an over-the-counter triple-antibiotic ointment twice a day, says Dr. Gigliotti. If the burn doesn't heal quickly or if it starts getting worse, call your vet right away.

Simple heat burns are usually the easiest to treat. Other types of burns, however, need more than a little bit of ice.

Chemical burns. These are caused by household cleaners or yard chemicals. "Flush the area with lots of water to wash away the chemical and stop further burns," says Dr. Gigliotti. Then take your pet to the vet immediately.

Electrical burns. A playful puppy or kitten will chew through almost anything, including electrical cords. This can cause a nasty burn around or inside the mouth. In more serious cases, electrical burns can damage lung tissue or even stop breathing entirely. Signs of lung injuries include coughing or difficulty breathing. Electrical burns are always an emergency that needs a veterinarian's care, says Dr. Gigliotti.

Car Accidents

Getting hit by a car is always an emergency, even if your pet gets up afterward and walks away, says Dr. Carter. There could be brain damage, internal bleeding, or nerve injuries that don't show up right away. Getting your pet to the vet soon after an accident could save her life.

In the meantime, here's what you can do to help.

1. Muzzle your pet before trying to move her. It's the only way to get her to safety without getting hurt yourself. (For more information, see "Muzzling an Injured Pet" on page 246.)
2. Check for breathing by looking at the rise and fall of her chest. You should also check her pulse by feeling the inside of the leg near the groin. If there is no pulse or she isn't breathing, start CPR immediately. (For instructions on administering CPR, see "Administering CPR" on page 249.)
3. Stop any bleeding by using a bandage, pushing on the pressure points, or, if necessary, applying a tourniquet.

(For more information, see "Stopping Bleeding" on page 248.)

4. Cover her with a blanket or coat to prevent shock.

5. If you suspect a bone is broken, splint the area to keep it immobile. (For more on splinting, see "Fractures" on page 257.)

6. Get her to a vet immediately.

Choking

Dogs tend to gobble as much food as they can as quickly as they can. And the quicker they gobble and swallow, the more likely they are to start choking. This is especially true for older dogs, which sometimes lose control over their swallowing reflexes.

Choking usually doesn't last very long. A few good "ack"s will often clear the windpipe of whatever is stuck inside. When the object doesn't come out, however, you need to act quickly. "Lacking enough oxygen, your pet may faint," says Dr. Carter. This means that the brain isn't getting enough oxygen. In a way, fainting is good, he adds. When your dog faints, it is easier to reach inside her mouth and remove whatever is causing the choking.

If you are unable to remove the object by hand, you may need to do the Heimlich maneuver. By pressing on her sides below the ribs, you will cause the diaphragm to push forward, creating pressure inside the airways. This will often "blow" the object right out, Dr. Carter explains. Here's the technique.

If your pet is standing. Stand behind your pet and wrap your arms tightly around her belly so they meet under the rib cage. (For cats and smaller dogs, grab the sides with your hands.) Make a fist with one hand and place your other hand over the fist. Then push up into the belly, giving your pet a quick, forceful squeeze. This will often pop the object right out. The smaller the pet, the more gently you should squeeze. If the object isn't dislodged with gentle force, gradually increase the force with each additional squeeze.

If your pet is unconscious. Lay her on her side. Feel for the last rib, near your pet's hindquarters. For cats and small dogs, place one hand over the shoulder blades to keep them steady. With the other hand, push behind the last rib and up into the abdomen five times. For dogs over 40 pounds, lie down behind her and wrap your arms around her abdomen. Make a fist with one hand and place your other hand over the fist. Press up into the abdomen five times, then check to see if the airway is clear. If not, try the abdominal press again.

Cuts

Pets often get cuts—not only on the pads of their paws but also on their legs and backs. Taking care of cuts right away will help ensure that minor cuts stay that way. "Cleaning wounds helps prevent infection and speeds healing," says Beverly J. Scott, D.V.M., a veterinarian in private practice in Gilbert, Arizona.

Begin by trimming the fur around the cut, advises Dr. Scott. Wash the area thoroughly with warm water. Rinse it well, then pat it dry with gauze pads. (Don't use cotton balls to dry a wound because the fibers will get stuck inside.) When the cut is clean, smear on some over-the-counter triple-antibiotic ointment several times a day.

Minor cuts usually don't need to be bandaged. In fact, they will heal a little faster when air is allowed to circulate. If your pet is licking or worrying the area, however, cover it up.

It is also a good idea to bandage cuts on the feet because the pads contain a lot of blood vessels that bleed easily. When bandaging a cut on a paw, start at the toes and wrap gauze around the paw and the lower part of the

Making a First-Aid Kit

Emergencies occur in a flash. Vets recommend always having a first-aid kit prepared and ready to go. Here's what to include.

- Your veterinarian's phone number
- The phone number of the closest emergency 24-hour clinic
- A first-aid manual, such as *The First-Aid Companion for Dogs and Cats* (Rodale, 2001)
- Antibacterial soap
- Antibiotic ointment
- Bandaging materials: 2-inch stretchable and nonstretchable gauze rolls; gauze pads in a variety of sizes
- Blunt-tipped scissors
- Cotton balls
- Disposable rubber gloves
- Hydrogen peroxide (3 percent)
- Masking tape
- Needle-nose pliers
- Petroleum jelly
- Plastic, needleless syringe or turkey baster
- Rectal thermometer
- Saline solution (for an eyewash)
- Tweezers

leg. Cover the gauze with overlapping strips of cloth bandage tape, making sure it isn't so tight that it cuts off circulation. If your pet is chewing at the dressing, put a sock over the foot and tape it in place.

Most cuts don't need anything more than this, says Dr. Scott. But if the cut is deep, longer than ½ inch, or packed with dirt, it is going to need a thorough cleaning, and you should call your vet.

Drowning

Dogs and cats are capable swimmers, but they tire easily, and once they are in the water, it isn't always easy for them to get out. They can drown very quickly if you aren't there to bail them out, says Dr. Trueba.

Veterinarians recommend covering swimming pools when they are not in use or at least putting a fence around the pool area. If you have kittens in the house, don't forget to keep the lid to the toilet closed. Young cats may jump up and fall in. The slippery sides of the toilet bowl make it difficult for them to get back out.

If your pet has somehow gotten into water and is unconscious or choking, move very quickly. Here is what Dr. Trueba advises.

1. Put your arms around her belly below the ribs and lift her into the air so that her torso is lower than her hips. (For heavy dogs, heft them from the rear and leave the front feet on the ground.) Gently swing her back and forth to shake water from the lungs.

2. Lay your pet on her side with her head slightly lower than her body. (If you are not on a hill, elevate her body by putting a towel or pillow beneath her back haunches.) This will allow additional water to drain from the lungs.

3. Check her pulse and breathing. If she isn't breathing, perform CPR immediately. If possible, have someone else call the vet while you continue to do CPR. (See "Administering CPR" on page 249.)

4. Get her to the vet as soon as possible.

Fractures

Mother Nature teaches pets to stay off an injured leg, especially a broken one, and they have "extra" legs that they can limp along on. But you still need to see the vet if your pet has a fractured bone, of course.

Unless the break is severe, it will probably be fairly easy to repair, says L. R. Danny Daniel, D.V.M., a veterinarian in private practice in Covington, Louisiana. There are two types of common leg fractures: those above the knee or elbow and those below. Those above the joints usually require orthopedic surgery to repair. Those below can often be stabilized with a splint alone. In either case, your pet will need to be kept quiet for 6 to 8 weeks in order for the fracture to heal properly.

Before taking your pet to the vet, it is important to stabilize a broken bone to prevent further damage. Here's how.

Fractures above the knee. Slide your pet onto a flat surface—a sturdy piece of cardboard, for example, or a small sheet of plywood—with the broken leg on the bottom. Tape the broken leg down with masking tape, then secure your pet's whole body to the board by covering her with a sheet or blanket and tying the ends together underneath the board. Then get her to the vet right away.

Fractures below the knee. Pad the leg with a towel to prevent chafing. Splint the leg using a pencil, a broken-off yardstick, or even a rolled-up magazine. The splint should extend from above the elbow or knee down to the bottom of the paw. Wrap it in place with gauze strips or bandage tape. Don't make it too tight, which could cut off bloodflow. Then get your pet to the vet.

Heatstroke

Heatstroke is an extremely serious condition in which a dog's or cat's internal temperature rises above 104°F, possibly causing damage to the brain or other organs. (Their normal temperature is between 100.5° and 102.5°F.) Short-faced breeds like pugs, boxers, and Persians, which have small airways, have an especially high risk of getting heatstroke. So do German shepherds, Old English sheepdogs, and other dogs with double coats, which retain a lot more heat than single coats.

"The leading cause of heatstroke in cats and dogs is leaving them in a parked car," says Lori A. Wise, D.V.M.,

Purging the Poison

When your pet has swallowed poison, vomiting is often the best way to get it out again. To induce vomiting, give a small amount of 3 percent hydrogen peroxide—about 1 teaspoon per 10 pounds of weight. Draw the liquid into a turkey baster or syringe and squirt it toward the back of your pet's mouth. Vomiting will usually occur within a few minutes. "If it doesn't work the first time, give the same amount in 15 to 20 minutes," advises Steve Hansen, D.V.M., vice president of the American Society for the Prevention of Cruelty to Animals' National Animal Poison Control Center in Urbana, Illinois. Don't use syrup of ipecac, however, because it can be toxic for dogs and cats.

Be aware that vomiting can make things worse with some poisons. Caustic substances like drain cleaner, for example, will do a "double burn"—once when your pet swallows them and again if she vomits them back up, Dr. Hansen adds.

Here are some common poisons, along with advice regarding whether or not to induce vomiting. Induce vomiting only if your pet is awake and alert. And get her to the vet pronto.

a veterinarian in private practice in Wheat Ridge, Colorado. Pets that are elderly or overweight or those that get too much vigorous exercise on a hot day can also get overheated. Signs of heatstroke include heavy panting and drooling, glassy eyes, deep-red gums, and excessive weakness.

Heatstroke is an emergency that must be treated by a vet, says Dr. Wise. In the meantime, you must act very quickly to bring the pet's temperature down. If possible,

Poison	Induce Vomiting
Antifreeze	Yes
Ant poison	Yes
Aspirin	Yes
Battery acid	No
Bleach	No
Drain cleaner	No
Fertilizer	No
Household cleaners	No
Insecticides	Yes
Medications (antihistamines, tranquilizers, barbiturates, amphetamines, heart pills, vitamins)	Yes
Paint thinner	No
Pesticides (water-based only)	Yes
Rodent poison	Yes
Sidewalk salt	No
Slug and snail bait	Yes
Turpentine	No
Weed killers (water-based only)	Yes
White glue or paste	No

immerse her entire body in cool (not cold) water in the bathtub, a child's swimming pool, or a laundry sink. If you are unable to get her all the way into the water, soak her with a garden hose or cover her with wet towels. (Dip the towels in cool water every 5 minutes.) It is also a good idea to put her in front of a fan or the air conditioner, preferably in the car while you are on your way to the vet.

Poisoning

Poisoning is always an emergency that requires *fast* veterinary care, says Steve Hansen, D.V.M., vice president of the American Society for the Prevention of Cruelty to Animals' National Animal Poison Control Center in Urbana, Illinois. But unless you actually see your pet eating something she shouldn't, you won't know right away that she has been poisoned. Symptoms to watch for include difficulty breathing, depression, confusion, seizures, a slow or fast heartbeat, excessive salivation, burns around the mouth, or bleeding from the nose, mouth, or anus.

If you suspect that your pet has been poisoned, call your vet or the animal poison control center immediately. (It's a good idea to write down these numbers ahead of time and put them on the refrigerator or in your first-aid kit.) Have the container of the suspected substance in front of you so that you can explain to the experts exactly what she got into, says Dr. Hansen.

Alternative-Healing Resource Guide

Natural and Holistic Veterinary Associations

You can send a self-addressed, stamped envelope to receive a list of practitioners in your area.

Academy of Veterinary Homeopathy
751 NE 168th Street
North Miami, FL 33162

American Academy of Veterinary Acupuncture
AAVA
P.O. Box 419
Hygiene, CO 80533-0419

American Holistic Veterinary Medical Association
2214 Old Emmorton Road
Bel Air, MD 21015

American Veterinary Chiropractic Association
623 Main Street
Hillsdale, IL 61257

Florida Holistic Veterinary Medical Association
751 Northeast 168th Street
North Miami Beach, FL 33162

Georgia Holistic Veterinary Medical Association
334 Knollwood Lane
Woodstock, GA 30188

Great Lakes Holistic Veterinary Medical Association (mostly Illinois and Wisconsin)
9824 Durand Avenue
Sturtevant, WI 53177

International Association for Veterinary Homeopathy
Sonnhaldenstr. 18
CH-8370 Sirnach
Switzerland

International Veterinary Acupuncture Society
P.O. Box 1478
Longmont, CO 80502

Rocky Mountain Holistic Veterinary Medical Association
311 South Pennsylvania Street
Denver, CO 80209

Natural Health Organizations

American Massage Therapy Association
820 Davis Street, Suite 100
Evanston, IL 60201

Canadian Herb Society
Van Dusen Botanical Display Garden
5251 Oak Street
Vancouver, British Columbia
Canada V6M 4H1

Flower Essence Society
P.O. Box 459
Nevada City, CA 95959

Office of Alternative Medicine Clearinghouse
National Institutes of Health
P.O. Box 8218
Silver Spring, MD 20907

Linda Tellington-Jones
TEAM and TTouch Trainings
P.O. Box 3793
Santa Fe, NM 87501

Publications

Best Friends Magazine
Best Friends Animal Sanctuary
5001 Angel Canyon Drive
Kanab, UT 84741

Dr. Bob and Susan Goldstein's Love of Animals Natural Care and Healing for Your Pets
606 Post Road East
Westport, CT 06880

The Enchanted Connections Review
18 Josephine Lane
Fort Salonga, NY 11768

Natural Cat and Dog
Fancy Publications
P.O. Box 6050
Mission Viejo, CA 92690

Natural Rearing Newsletter
Ambrican Enterprises Ltd.
P.O. Box 1436
Jacksonville, OR 97530

North Star's Healthy Pets Naturally!
148 Channel Road
Tinmouth, VT 05773

PetSage
4313 Wheeler Avenue
Alexandria, VA 22304

Aromatherapy and Essential Oils

Aura Cacia
P.O. Box 399
Weaverville, CA 96093

Oshadhi USA
1340 G. Industrial Avenue
Petaluma, CA 94952

Young Living Essential Oils
250 South Main Street
Payson, UT 84651

Flower Essences

Alaskan Flower Essence Project
P.O. Box 1369
Homer, AK 99603
Specializes in flower, gem, and environmental essences.

Flower Essences Services
P.O. Box 1769
Nevada City, CA 95959

Global Health Alternatives
193 Middle Street, Suite 201
Portland, ME 04101

Green Hope Farm Flower Essences
P.O. Box 125
Meriden, NH 03770

The Source
2501 71st Street
North Bergen, NJ 07047
Specializes in flower remedies.

Glandulars, Nutriceuticals, and Supplements

The Botanical Animal
Equilite, Inc.
20 Prospect Avenue
Ardsley, NY 10502

Natural Animal Nutrition
2109 Emmorton Park Drive
Edgewood, MD 21040

Nutramax Laboratories, Inc.
5024 Campbell Boulevard
Baltimore, MD 21236

Nutritech Inc.
5000 West Oakey Boulevard
Unit D-13
Las Vegas, NV 89146

Nutrition Now, Inc.
6350 Northeast Campus Drive
Vancouver, WA 98661

Prozyme Products Ltd.
6600 North Lincoln Avenue
Lincolnwood, IL 60645

Vita Plus Industries, Inc.
953 East Sahara Avenue
Suite 21B
Las Vegas, NV 89104

Herbs

Animals' Apawthecary
P.O. Box 212
Conner, MT 59827
Specializes in glycerine-based herbal preparations.

Azmira Holistic Animal Care
2100 N. Wilmot Road
Suite 109
Tucson, AZ 85712
Specializes in Western herbs.

Essiac International
P.O. Box 23155
Ottawa, Ontario
Canada K2A 4E2

Essiac (U.S. distributor)
3869 Mallard Way
Little River, SC 29566
Specializes in Essiac tea.

Frontier Natural Products Co-op
3021 78th Street
P.O. Box 299
Norway, IA 52318

Harmany Veterinary Products
3065 Center Green Drive
Suite 140
Boulder, CO 80301

Healing Herbs for Pets
4292-99 Fourth Avenue
Ottawa, Ontario
Canada K1S 5B3
Specializes in Chinese herbal remedies for dogs and cats.

Herb Pharm
P.O. Box 116
Williams, OR 97544
Specializes in organic herbs and tinctures.

Herb Research Foundation
1007 Pearl Street, Suite 200
Boulder, CO 80302

Merritt Naturals
P.O. Box 532
Rumson, NJ 07760

Homeopathic Remedies

Arnica, Inc.
144 East Garry Avenue
Santa Ana, CA 92707

Boiron
P.O. Box 559
6 Campus Boulevard, Building A
Newtown Square, PA 19073

Dr. Goodpet
P.O. Box 4547
Inglewood, CA 90309
Specializes in combination homeopathic remedies.

Dolisos America, Inc.
3014 Rigel Avenue
Las Vegas, NV 89102

Hahnemann Laboratories, Inc.
1940 Fourth Street
San Rafael, CA 94901

Heel BHI
11600 Cochiti Road Southeast
Albuquerque, NM 87123

Homeopathic Educational Services
2124 Kittredge Street
Berkeley, CA 94704

Standard Homeopathic Company
154 West 131st Street
Los Angeles, CA 90061

Index

Underscored page references indicate boxed text.